Alternative Therapy Health Series

Herbal Cure

Medicinal Plants that Heal Naturally

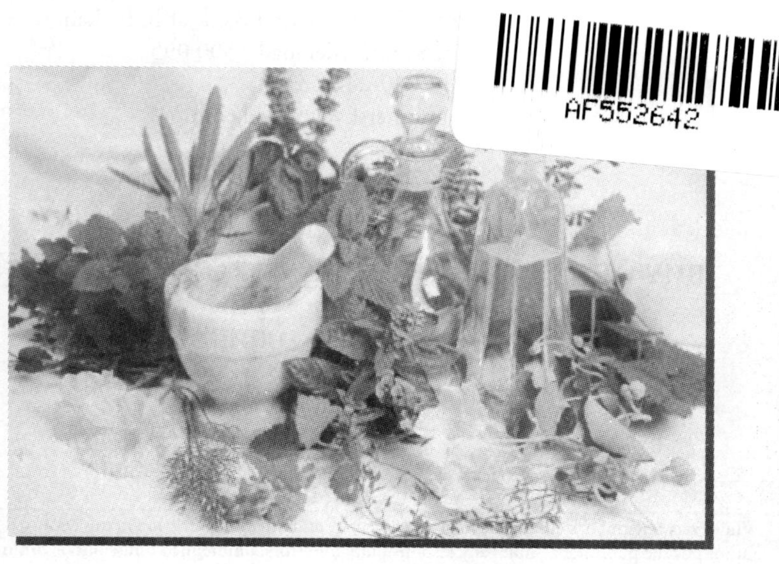

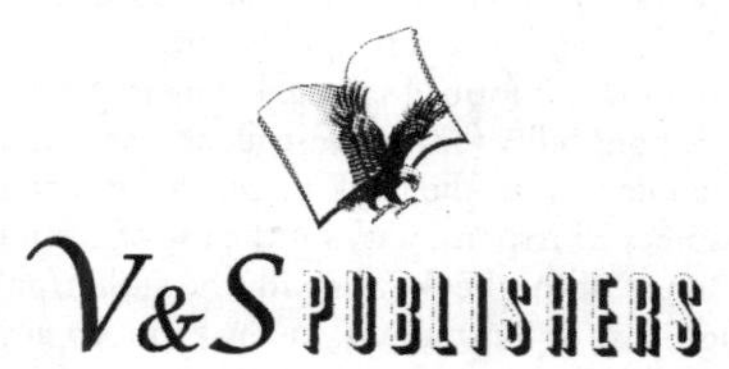

Published by:

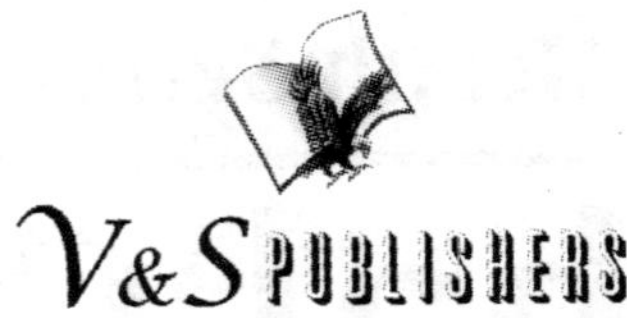

F-2/16, Ansari road, Daryaganj, New Delhi-110002
☎ 23240026, 23240027 • *Fax:* 011-23240028
info@vspublishers.com • www.vspublishers.com

Online Brandstore: amazon.in/vspublishers

Regional Office : Hyderabad
5-1-707/1, Brij Bhawan (Beside Central Bank of India Lane)
Bank Street, Koti, Hyderabad - 500 095
☎ 040-24737290
vspublishershyd@gmail.com

Follow us on: 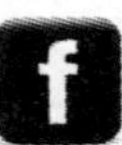 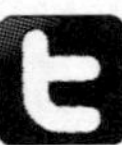 

BUY OUR BOOKS FROM: AMAZON FLIPKART

ISBN 978-93-505718-4-2
New Edition

DISCLAIMER

While every attempt has been made to provide accurate and timely information in this book, neither the author nor the publisher assumes any responsibility for errors, unintended omissions or commissions detected therein. The author and publisher make no representation or warranty with respect to the comprehensiveness or completeness of the contents provided.

All matters included have been simplified under professional guidance for general information only without any warranty for applicability on an individual. Any mention of an organization or a website in the book by way of citation or as a source of additional information doesn't imply the endorsement of the content either by the author or the publisher. It is possible that websites cited may have changed or removed between the time of editing and publishing the book.

Results from using the expert opinion in this book will be totally dependent on individual circumstances and factors beyond the control of the author and the publisher.

It makes sense to elicit advice from well informed sources before implementing the ideas given in the book. The reader assumes full responsibility for the consequences arising out from reading this book. For proper guidance, it is advisable to read the book under the watchful eyes of parents/guardian. The purchaser of this book assumes all responsibility for the use of given materials and information.

Printed at : Param Offsetters, Okhla, New Delhi–110020

Publisher`s Note

Medicinal Plants and Herbs have been used by mankind from times immemorial, particularly in the traditional Indian systems of medicine, such as *Ayurveda* and *Homeopathy*. Some of them are even toxic, but of immense pharmaceutical value.

Basically, plants have the ability to synthesise a wide variety of chemical compounds that are used to perform important biological functions and to defend against attack from predators, like insects, fungi, bacteria and viruses, thus, protecting us from a number of deadly diseases like Cancer, Tuberculosis, AIDS and many incurable Skin and Venereal diseases.

The study of plants for medicinal purposes is called as *Herbalism* or *Herbal Medicine* and the usage of these medicinal plants for treatment and cure of different types of diseases is known as ***Herbal Cure***. This book contains an *exhaustive list of about 130 medicinal plants and herbs* which are used totally or in parts, such as their roots, stems, leaves, or barks, crushed or decocted, boiled or mixed with water or honey, etc., to treat innumerable commonly occurring diseases like: cough and cold, fevers, pneumonia, skin diseases, indigestion, diarrhoea, asthma, and even snake-bites and scorpion-stings.

Though all the usage and treatments suggested in the book have been authenticated by the author, yet a doctor's advice is a must before consuming or applying these plant extracts on your body.

All said and done, the book has been aimed to enlighten all its readers about the *Natural Cure and Healing of several diseases with Plants and Plant Products, which generally do not have any side effects and help to completely eradicate the diseases from their roots*. Hope the book is beneficial to all and serves its purpose well. We would be glad to receive your valuable suggestions and queries on the subject to make it all the more appealing and worth reading..............

However, though all the treatments suggested in the book have been authenticated by the author, yet a doctor's advice is a must before consuming or applying these plant extracts on your body.

Contents

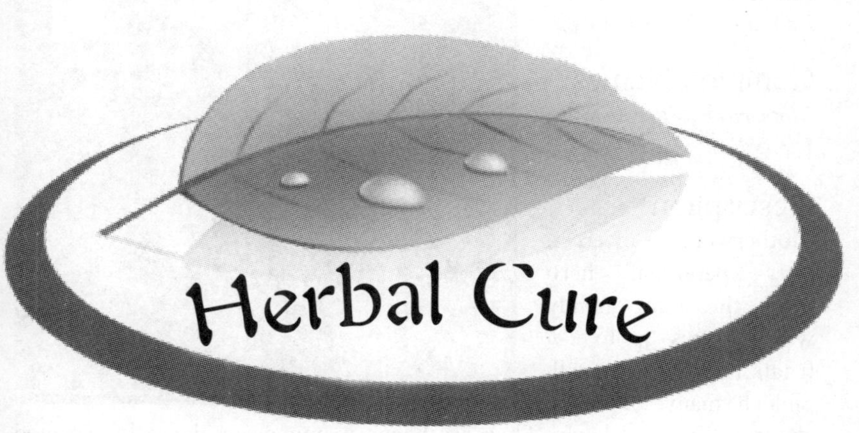
Herbal Cure

Motherwort

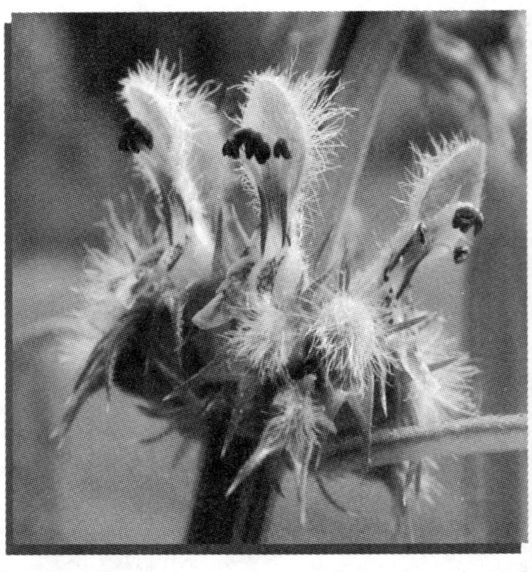

Botanical Name
Leonurus cardiaca

Family
Lamiaceae (Mint family)

Common Names
Motherwort, Throw-wort, Lion's Ear

Description
Motherwort is an erect, leafy perennial herb from the mint family which grows up to 2-5 ft tall. Flowers are small, pinkish, mauve or white, about 1.2 cm and hairy. They are borne in numerous dense interrupted whorls, in leafy spikes. Flowers are two-lipped, upper concave, and the lower 3-lobed. Leaves are ovate to lance-shaped, variously cut, but mostly with 3-7 deep or shallow triangular, toothed lobes. The upper leaves may be entire or 3-lobed. Motherwort is found in the Himalayas, from Pakistan to Nepal, at altitudes of 2400-3600 m. Flowering: June-August.

Medicinal Uses
Motherwort is primarily a herb of the heart. Several species have sedative effects, decreasing muscle spasms and temporarily lowering the blood pressure. Chinese studies found that the extracts from decrease clotting and the level of fat in the blood and can slow heart palpitations and rapid heartbeats. Another of motherwort's uses is to *improve fertility* and *reduce anxiety* associated with *childbirth, postpartum depression* and *menopause.* If used in early labour, it, will *ease the labour pains* and *calm the nerves after childbirth.*

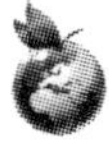

Honeyweed

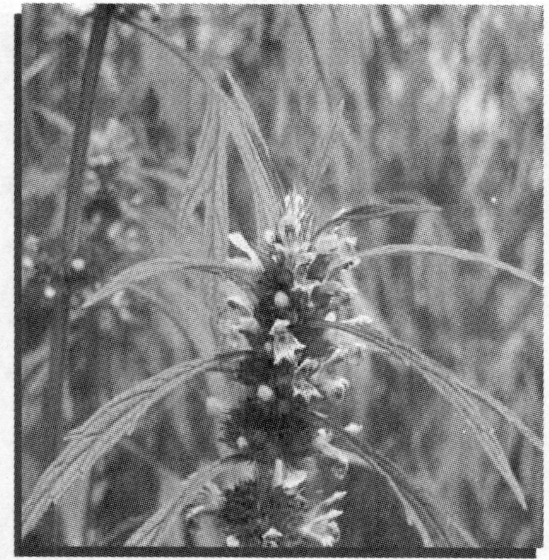

Botanical Name
Leonurus japonicus

Family
Lamiaceae (Mint family)

Synonyms
Leonurus sibiricus

Common Names
Honeyweed, Chinese Motherwort, Little marijuana

Description
Honeyweed is an east Asian relative of motherwort, a well-known European weed used traditionally to treat infections and circulatory and menstruation disorders. Chinese motherwort grows in the first summer 4-5 ft high and flowers from August until late fall. The flowers and the fine foliage resembling Japanese maples are quite pretty and would make a nice herb garden hedge, but the branches get bare and twiggy in late summer. Whilst flowering continues, the leaves turn reddish and fall off in late September.

Medicinal Uses
It is known in *Chinese medicine* as *Yi-mu-cao.* The *Chinese motherwort* is unusual amongst the Chinese herbs in that it is often prescribed for use on its own and not in a mixture with other plants. The whole plant is *antibacterial, antispasmodic, astringent, cardiac, depurative, diaphoretic, diuretic, emmenagogue, hypnotic, nervine, oxytocic, stomachic, tonic, uterine stimulant.*

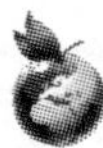

Common Leucas

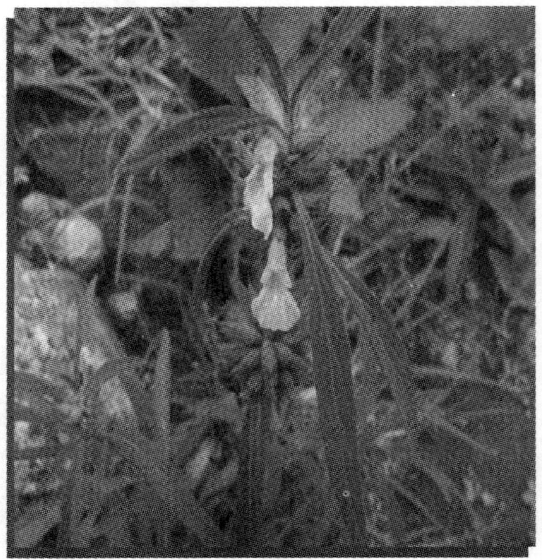

Botanical Name:
Leucas aspera

Family
Lamiaceae (Mint family)

Common Names
Common Leucas • Hindi: *Chhota halkusa, Gophaa* • Manipuri: *Mayanglambum* • Marathi: *Tamba* • Tamil: *Thumbai* • Malayalam: *Tumba* • Telugu: *Tummachettu* • Kannada: *Tumbe guda* • Bengali: *Ghal ghase* • Oriya: *Bhutamari* • Konkani: *Tumbo* • Sanskrit: *Dronapushpi*

Description
Common Leucas is an erect and diffusely branched annual herb. Leaves are linear or oblong, 2.5 to 7.5 cm long with blunt tips and scalloped margins. Whorls are large, terminal and axillary, about 2.5 cm in diameter and crowded with white bell shaped flowers. *Calyx is variable, with an upper lip and short, triangular teeth.*

Medicinal Uses
A popular Pot Herb believed to help develop resistance to fight diseases.

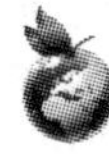

Horse Mint

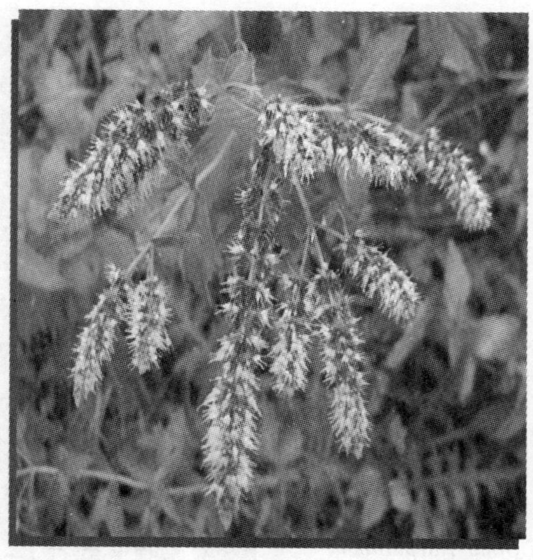

Botanical Name
Mentha longifolia

Family
Lamiaceae (Mint family)

Common Names
Horse Mint, Habek Mint, Biblical Mint, Cow-weed

Description
Horse Mint is an aromatic, perennial herb with stem erect, leaves lanceolate, ovate or oblong, tooth, nearly sessile arranged opposite on the stem. The unusual long, narrow leaves of Habek Mint are true to its Latin name, *longifolia.* Flowers are small, lilac in whorls forming slender spike often interrupted below, borne at the ends of branches and forming a lax densely hairy inflorescence. Flowers are hairy outside. Bracts lanceolate. Sepals sharply 5- toothed, bell shaped, petals 4- lobed, lobes erect, stamen 4, exerted. Fruit, nutlet.

Medicinal Uses
The *infusion of leaves* is taken as a cooling medicine. *Dried leaves* and *flowers tops are carminative* and *stimulant.* It is believed to the best remedy for headaches.

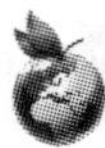

Bengal Sage

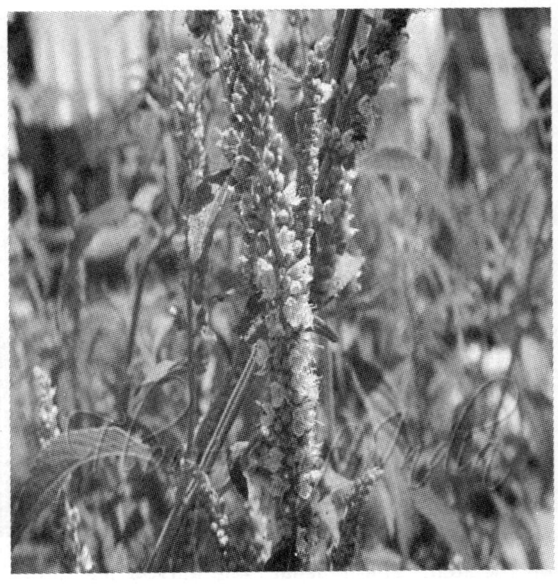

Botanical Name:
Meriandra benghalensis

Family:
Lamiaceae **(Mint family)**

Synonyms:
Salvia bengalensis

Common Names:
Bengal Sage, Bengali *Salvia* • Hindi: *Kafur-ka pat* • Manipuri: *Kanghu-maan* • Tamil: *Chayayilai* • Telugu: *Sima-Karpuramu* • Bengali: *Kafur-ka pat*

Description:
Bengal Sage is a herb from the mint family. It has elliptic-oblong green leaves with serrated margins. Tiny while flowers arise on a long vertical spike, much like that in Tulsi. The herb is cultivated for medicinal uses.

Medicinal Uses:
Fresh leaves are given for reducing high blood pressure. *Extracts of inflorescences is used as gargle in tonsilitis.*

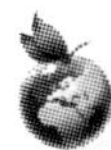

Catnip

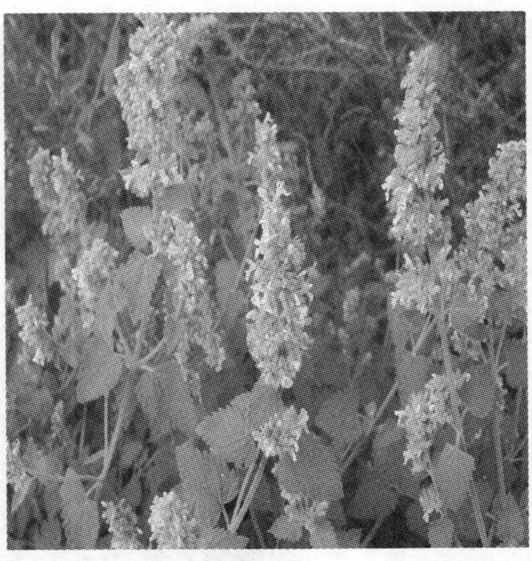

Botanical Name:

Nepeta cataria

Family:

Lamiaceae **(Mint family)**

Common Names:

Catnip, Catmint

Description:

Catnip and catmints are mainly known for, and named after, the effects they have on cats, particularly domestic cats. Catnip contains nepetalactone, a terpene, that is thought to mimic feline sex pheromones. Cats detect it through their vomeronasal organs. When cats sense the bruised leaves or stems of catnip, they will rub in it, roll over it, paw at it, chew it, lick it, leap about and purr. Catnip is a 50–100 cm tall herb resembling mint in appearance, with hairy green leaves; the flowers are white, with purple markings. They have sturdy stems with opposite heart-shaped, green to greyish-green leaves. The flowers are white and occur in several clusters towards the tip of the stems. Before the introduction of Chinese tea, catmint was used to make tea by the British.

Medicinal Uses:

Due to the fact that catnip *promotes sweating* when used as an *herbal tea*, it was used for the treatment of *nervousness, colds, influenza* and fevers during the Middle Ages. Catnip has also been alleged to aid with *flatulence, diarrhoea, colic* and other *childhood diseases*, as well as *preventing miscarriages, premature births,* and *morning sicknesses.*

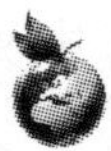

Pink Catmint

Botanical Name:
Nepeta spp.

Family:
Lamiaceae **(Mint family)**

Common Names:
Catnip, Pink Catmint

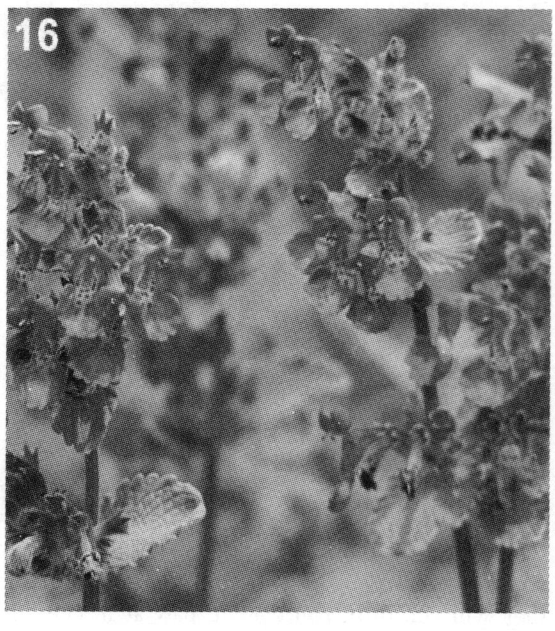

Description:
Pink Catmint, a cousin of the better known *Nepeta cataria,* is a 50–100 cm tall herb resembling mint in appearance, with hairy green leaves; the flowers are pinkish white, with purple throat.

The genus is native to Europe, Asia and Africa, with the highest species diversity in the Mediterranean region east to China. Most of the species are herbaceous perennial plants, but some are annuals.

They have sturdy stems with opposite heart-shaped, green to greyish-green leaves. The flowers are white, blue, pink or lilac and occur in several clusters toward the tip of the stems. Before the introduction of Chinese tea, *catmint was used to make tea by the British.*

Catnip and catmints are mainly known for, and named after, the effects they have on cats, particularly domestic cats. Catnip contains nepetalactone, a terpene, that is thought to mimic feline sex pheromones.

Cats detect it through their vomeronasal organs. When cats sense the bruised leaves or stems of catnip, they will rub in it, roll over it, paw at it, chew it, lick it, leap about and purr.

Medicinal Uses:

Due to the fact that *catnip promotes sweating* when used as an *herbal tea*, it was used for the treatment of *nervousness, colds, influenza* and *fevers* during the Middle Ages.

Catnip has also been alleged to aid with *flatulence, diarrhoea, colic* and other *childhood diseases*, as well as preventing *miscarriages, premature births,* and *morning sickness.*

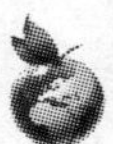

Tulsi

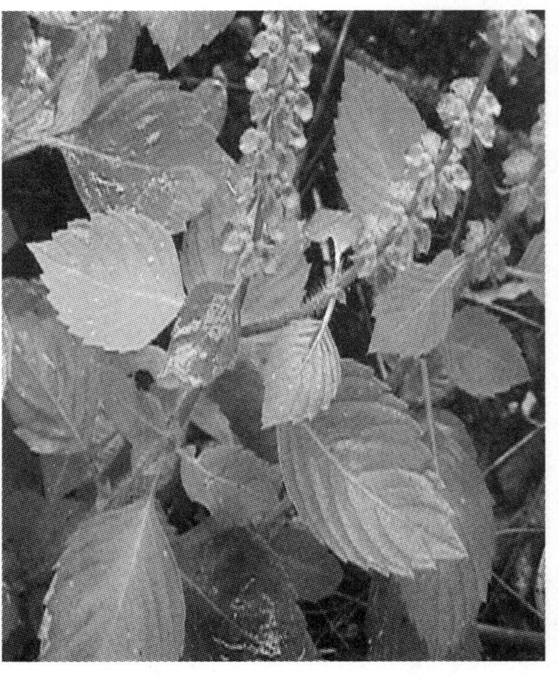

Botanical Name:
Ocimum sanctum

Family:
Lamiaceae **(Mint family)**

Common Names:
Holy basil • Hindi, Tamil, Telugu: *Tulsi* • Malayalam: *Trittavu* • Marathi: *Tulshi*

Description:
Tulsi (Ocimum sanctum) is a widely grown, sacred plant of India. Hindus grow Tulsi as a religious plant in their homes, temples and their farms.

They use *Tulsi* leaves in routine worship. *Tulsi*, grown as a pot plant, is found in almost every traditional Hindu house.

The natural habitat of *Tulsi* varies from sea level to an altitude of 2000 m. It is found growing naturally in moist soil nearly all over the globe. Tulsi is a branched, fragrant and erect herb having hair all over. It attains a height of about 75 to 90 cm when mature. Its leaves are nearly round and up to 5 cm long with the margin being entire or toothed.

These are aromatic because of the presence of a kind of scented oil in them. A variety with green leaves is called *Shri* Tulsi and one with reddish leaves is called *Krishna Tulsi*.

Tulsi flowers are small having purple to reddish colour, present in small compact clusters on cylindrical spikes. The fruits are small and the seeds yellow to reddish in colour.

Medicinal Uses:

Because of its *medicinal virtues*, Tulsi is used in *Ayurvedic preparations* for *treating various ailments.*

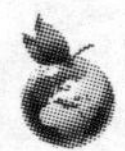

Cat`s Whiskers

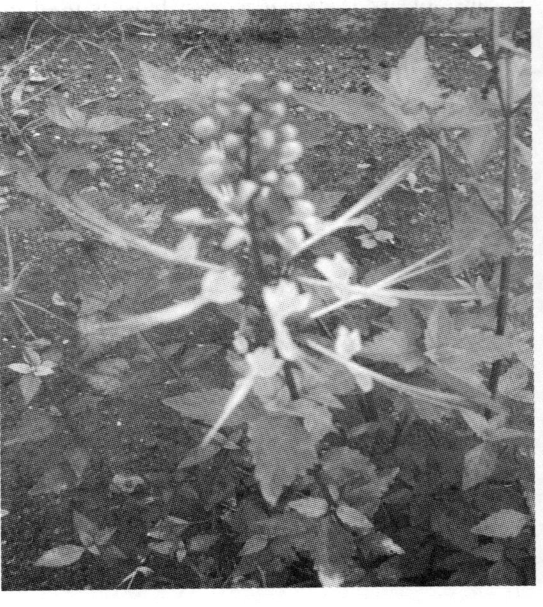

Botanical Name:
Orthosiphon aristatus

Family:
Lamiaceae **(Mint family)**

Synonyms:
Clerodendrum spicatum, Orthosiphon spiralis, Orthosiphon stamineus

Common Names:
Cat's Whiskers, Java Tea, Kidney Tea Plant • Manipuri: *Warak Leikham* • Mizo: *Zunthlum-kung*

Description:
Cat's Whiskers is a perennial herb found mainly throughout South-east Asia and tropical Australia. It grows to be about 1 to 3 feet tall and has a very open branching habit with 1-inch dark green, ovate leaves with serrated margins. At the end of the branches are racemes of flowers. When the flowers open, the stamens and pistil extend out far beyond the petals, creating the 'cat's whiskers' effect. The flowers are most commonly white, but they can also occur in light shades of purple.

Medicinal Uses:
In Manipur, the leaves are used as tea in *kidney and bladder diseases.* According to clinical studies, infusion of dried leaf has *diuretic effect* and increases the *uric acid excretion.*

Cuban Oregano

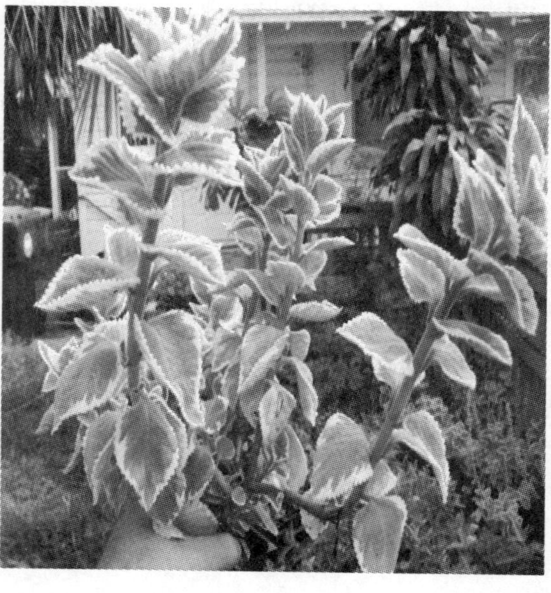

Botanical Name:
Plectranthus amboinicus

Family:
Lamiaceae **(Mint family)**

Synonyms:
Coleus amboinicus, Coleus aromaticus, Plectranthus aromaticus

Common Names:
Cuban Oregano, Indian borage, Indian mint, Mexican mint, Mexican oregano, Spanish thyme • Hindi: *Patharchur, Patta ajwain* • *Marathi: Pathurchur* • Tamil: *Karpuravalli* • Malayalam: *Panikkurkka, Kannikkurkka* • Telugu: *Sugandhavalkam, Karpoora valli, Karuvaeru, Vamu aaku* • Kannada: *Karpurahalli, Dodda pathre, Dodda pathre soppu, Karpoora valli* • Sanskrit: *Karpuravalli, Sugandhavalakam*

Description:
Cuban Oregano is a sprawling and somewhat succulent herb, growing to 1 m tall. The plant is sometimes prostrate at base, with the branchlets rising up, densely hairy. Leaves have stalks 1-4.5 cm long, densely velvety, like most mint family plants.

Leaf blade is fleshy, broadly ovate to circular, rhombic, or kidney-shaped, 4-10 cm long, 3-9 cm broad, coarsely toothed at margin or entire toward base. Flowers are borne in 10-20-flowered, densely velvety spikes, 10-20 cm long.

Flower stalks are slender, up to 5 mm long. Sepal cup is bell-shaped, 1.5-4 mm long. Flowers are pale blue or mauve to pink, 8-12 mm long - the upper lip is up to 4.5 x 3 mm, erect, the lower lip up to 5-6 x 4 mm, concave. Filaments of stamens are mostly fused into a tube around style. The origin of Cuban Oregano is unknown - it is widely cultivated world-wide. The leaves are strongly flavoured and make an excellent addition to stuffings for meat and poultry. Finely chopped, they can also be used to flavour meat dishes, especially beef, lamb and game.

Medicinal Uses:

The *leaves* have also had many traditional medicinal uses, especially for the treatment of *coughs, sore throats and nasal congestion*, but also for a range of other problems, such as *infections*, *rheumatism* and *flatulence*. In Indonesia, the Cuban Oregano is a *traditional food* used in *soups* to stimulate *lactation* for the *month or so following childbirth.*

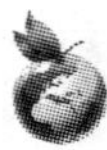

Sangbrei

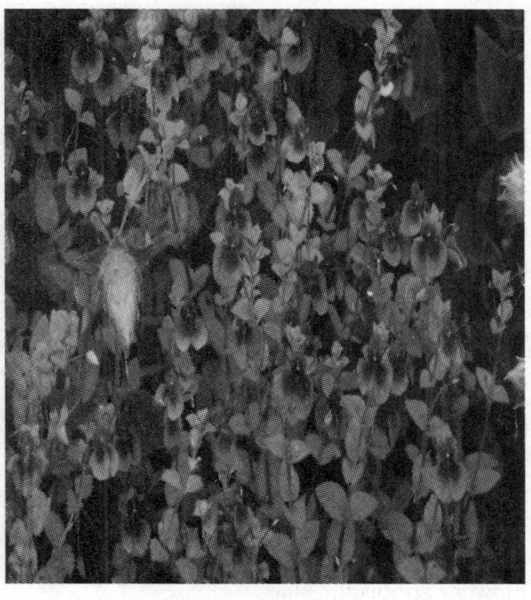

Botanical Name:
Pogostemon purpurascens

Family:
Lamiaceae **(Mint family)**

Common Names:
Sangbrei • Manipuri: Sangbrei, Shangbrei

Description:
Sangbrei is an erect or sub erect branched herbs, to 20 cm tall, with strong odour. Stem is 4-angled and hairy. Hairs are long, spreading, and sometimes glandular. Leaves occur in unequal, opposite pairs. Leaves are elliptic, with serrated margin, narrow tip and wedge-shaped base. Tiny whitish flowers, 6 mm long, are borne in elongated spikes. The stalk of the spike is up to 8 cm long. Bracts are 6 mm long, ovate-lanceshaped. Sepal tube is up to 4 mm long, hairy outside. It has lanceshaped, 3-nerved teeth. Flowers are 2-lipped - tube is narrow, about 5 mm long. Upper lip is 3-lobed, purplish, and the lower one entire. Stamens are 4 in number, protruding out. Style is long, slender, with a 2-lobed stigma - lobes are long, slender. In Manipur, leaves and flowers are used in the preparation of a local hair-care lotion. Flowering: January-February.

Medicinal Uses:
Leaves are *styptic* and used to *clean wounds* and for *promoting granulation.* Roots are used in *uterine haemorrhage, snake-bites* and *scorpion stings. Leaf juice is given in fever.*

Common Self-Heal

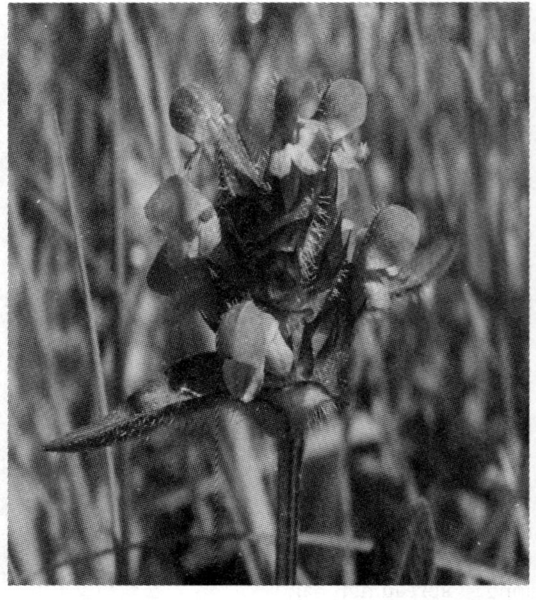

Botanical Name:

Prunella vulgaris var. vulgaris

Family:

Lamiaceae **(Mint family)**

Common Names:

Common Self-Heal, Heal-all, Heart-of-the-earth

Description:

Common Self-Heal is a herb found on the meadows and open slopes of the Himalayas, from Afghanistan to Bhutan. Flowers are bright blue-violet, rarely pink or white, up to 1.5 cm long.

They are borne in whorls of 6. Flowers are 2-lipped and tubular, the top lip is a purple hood, and the bottom lip has three lobes with the middle lobe being larger and fringed. Sepal cup is also tubular and 2-lipped, with a purplishtinge of colour. The inflorscence contains many purplish overlapping bracts. Stems are 10-30 cm long, creeping or rising.

Leaves are ovate or ovate-oblong, 1.5-6 × 0.7-2.5 cm. There is a pair of leaves just below the inflorescence.

Common Self-Heal is found at altitudes of 1500-3600 m. Common Self-Heal was once proclaimed to be a *holy herb* and was thought to be sent by God to cure all ailments of man or beast. It was said to drive away the devil, which lead to the belief that Heal-All was grown in the Witches garden as a disguise.

The root was also used to make a tea to drink in ceremonies before going hunting by one Native American tribe to sharpen the powers of observation.

[Flowering: May-September.

Medicinal Uses:

Heal-all is both *edible and medicinal.* It can be used in *salads, soups, stews,* or boiled as a *pot herb.* It has been used as an alternative medicine for centuries on just about every continent in the world, and for just about every ailment.

Heal-All is something of a panacea, and it does seem to have some medicinal uses that are constant. It is taken internally as a *medicinal tea* in *the treatment of fevers, diarrhoea, sore mouth and throat, internal bleeding and weaknesses of the liver and heart.*

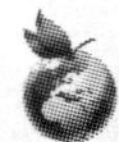

Bicolor Skullcap

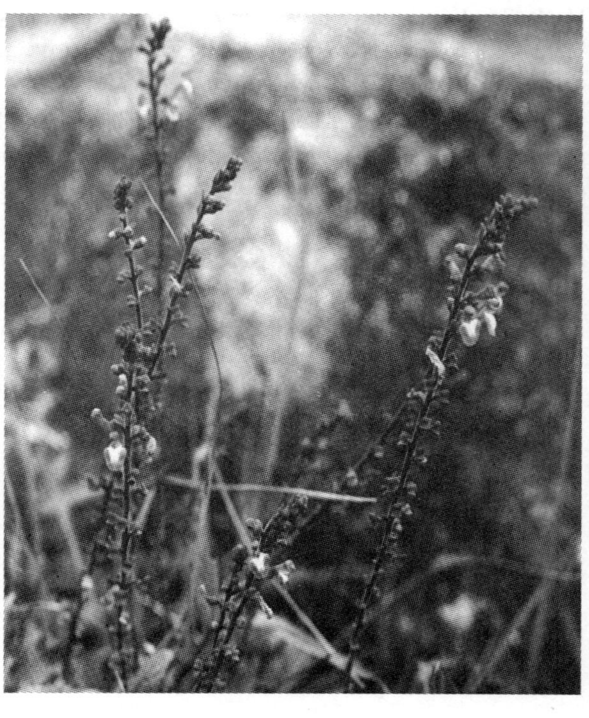

Botanical Name:
Scutellaria discolor

Family:
Lamiaceae **(Mint family)**

Synonyms:
Scutellaria indica

Common Names:
Bicolor Skullcap • Manipuri: *Yenakha* • Nepali: *Nilo butte* ghans, Daampaate

Description:
Bicolor Skullcap is a perennial shrub, with 1 to few stems, 1-2 ft tall. Flowers are blue, tubular 2-lipped, in long slender loose leafless spikes, 8-25 cm long.

Flowers are 1.3-1.8 cm long, with a slender, curved tube, opening into two lips. Upper lips is entire, hooded, and the lower one is broad, 3-lobed, often paler in colour. Sepals cup is 2 mm long, enlarging in fruit and covering the nutlets.

The Common Names of the plant comes from the sepal cups which look like medieval helmets. Elliptic leaves are mostly at the base, with blunt-toothed margins, 2-8 cm long, long stalked, often purple on the underside.

Bicolour Skullcap is found on shady banks in the Himalayas, from Uttarakhand to NE India, at altitudes of 700-2400 m. Flowering: July-November.

Medicinal Uses:

The juice of the plant is applied to wounds between the toes caused by prolonged walking barefooted in muddy water during the rainy season. *The juice of the root*, about four teaspoons twice a day, is given to treat *indigestion and gastric troubles.*

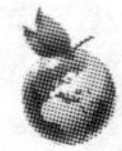

Barringtonia

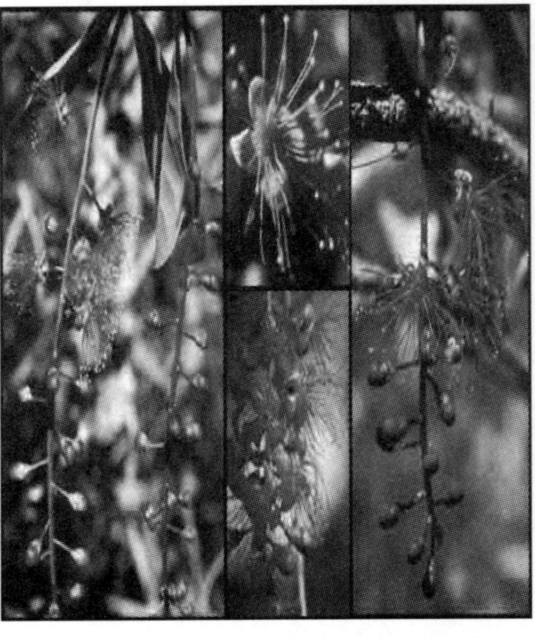

Botanical Name:
Barringtonia acutangula

Family:
Lecythidaceae **(Brazilnut family)**

Synonyms:
Barringtonia spicata, Eugenia acutangula

Common Names:
Barringtonia, Freshwater Mangrove, Indian Oak, Indian Putat • Assamese: *Hendol, Hinyol, Pani amra* • Bengali: *Hijal* • Hindi: *Hijagal, Hijjal, Samundarphal* • Kannada: *Mavinkubia, Niruganigily, Dhatripala* • Malayalam: *Attampu, Attupelu, Nir perzha* • Marathi: *Tiwar, Newar, Sathaphala, Samudraphala* • Oriya: *Nijhira* • Sanskrit: *Abdhiphala, Ambudhiphala, Ambuja* • Tamil: *Aram, Kadambu, Kadappai, Samudra pazham* • Telugu: *Kurpa* • Urdu: *Samandarphal*

Description:
Barringtonia is an evergreen tree of moderate size, called by Sanskrit writers Hijja or Hijjala. T

he fruit is spoken of as Samudra-phala and or the 'nurse's fruit,' and is one of the best known domestic remedies. Also called *Stream Barringtonia* or *Itchy Tree* (after a catepillar with irritant hairs that sometimes colonises the undersides of the leaves) Barringtonia is a tree 5-8 m tall with rough fissured dark grey bark.

Leaves are obovate. Red flowers are produced on pendulous racemes about 20cm long. Four sided fruits are produced periodically throughout the year.

Partly deciduous in extended dry periods. This species grows on the banks of freshwater rivers, the edges of freshwater swamps and lagoons and on seasonally flooded lowland plains, commonly on heavy soils. Found in Madagascar and tropical Asia, amongst other places. Propagation is by seed. Tolerant of heavy clay soils with poor drainage, it can grow in a range of soils.

Medicinal Uses:

This tree has long been used for *medicine, timber and as a fish poison.* In *traditional medicine,* when children suffer *from a cold in the chest, the seed is rubbed down on a stone with water* and applied *over the sternum,* and if there is much *dyspnoea,* a *few grains with or without the juice of fresh ginger are administered internally.* These seldom fail to induce vomiting and the expulsion of mucus from the air passages.

More recently, it has become the *focus of research for pain-killing compounds.*

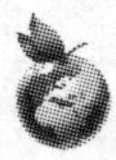

Wild Guava

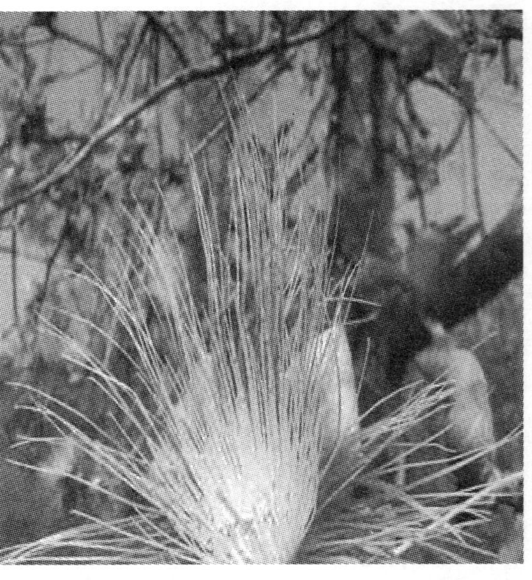

Botanical Name:
Careya arborea

Family:
Lecythidaceae (**Brazilnut Family**)

Common Names:
Wild Guava, Ceylon Oak, Patana Oak • Hindi: *Kumbhi*• Marathi: *Kumbha* • Tamil: *Aima, Karekku, Puta-tanni-maram* • Malayalam: *Alam, Paer, Peelam, Pela* • Telugu: *Araya, Budatadadimma, Budatanevadi, Buddaburija* • Kannada: *Alagavvele, Daddal* • Bengali: *Vakamba, Kumhi, Kumbhi* • Oriya: *Kumbh* • Khasi: *Ka Mahir, Soh Kundur* • Assamese: *Godhajam, Kum, Kumari, Kumbhi* • Sanskrit: *Bhadrendrani, Girikarnika, Kaidarya, Kalindi*

Description:
Wild Guava is a medium sized deciduous tree, up to 20 m tall, the leaves of which turn red in the cold season. It is the *Kumbhi* of Sanskrit writers, and appears to have been so named on account of the hollow on the top of the fruit giving it somewhat the appearance of a *water-pot.*

Wild pigs are very fond of the bark, and that it is used by hunters to attract them. An astringent gum exudes from the fruit and stem, and the bark is made into coarse cordage.

The Tamil name *Puta-tanni-maram* signifies 'water- bark-tree,' in allusion to the exudation trickling down the bark in dry weather. Bark surface flaking in thin strips, fissured, dark grey; crown spreading. Leaves are arranged spirally, often clustered at the apices of twigs, simple, broadly obovate, tapering at base, margin toothed, stipules small, caducous. Flowers in an erect raceme at the end of branches.

Flowers are large, white. Sepals are 4, petals 4, free. Stamens are many, connate at base; disk annular; ovary inferior, 4–5-locular with many ovules in 2 rows per cell, style 1. Fruit a large, many-seeded drupe, globose to depressed globose, crowned by the persistent sepals. Seedling with hypogeal germination; cotyledons absent (seed containing a swollen hypocotyl); shoot with scales at the first few nodes.

Medicinal Uses:

The *bark of the tree* and the *sepals of the flowers* are well-known *Indian remedies*, and are valued on account of their *astringent and mucilaginous properties*, it is also being administered internally in *coughs and colds* and applied externally as an embrocation.

Banchalita

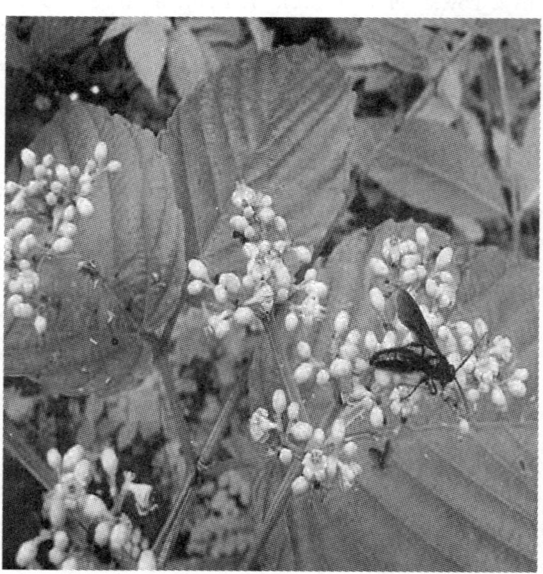

Botanical Name:
Leea asiatica

Family:
Leeaceae **(Leea family)**

Synonyms:
Leea aspera, Leea crispa, Phytolacca asiatica

Common Names:
Banchalita • Hindi: *Banchalita* • Manipuri: *Koknal* • Bengali: *Banchalita*

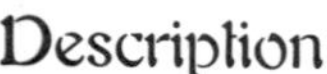

Description:
Banchalita is an erect gergarious shrub with angular stem swollen above the nodes and internodes. Petioles and peduncles usually have narrow crisped wings. Leaves are pinnately compound - not double-pinnate like Bandicoot Berry. Leaflets are 3-5, laterals opposite, ovate or ovate-oblong, serrate, tip sharp, base rounded or heart-shaped. Flowers, 5-6 mm across, greenish white, are borne in short, cymes at the end of branches. Calyx united, cup-like, teeth 5, obscure, often glandular-tipped. Petals 5, connate, 2-3 mm long, ovate, acute. Stamens 5, united; staminal tube 5-lobes, 2-celled. Ovary inserted on the disc; style short; stigma 2-lobed. Leaf extract is mixed with water and used for washing hair by Chiru tribe in NE India. Flowering: September.

Medicinal Uses:
Root tuber is used against *guineaworms.* The root with bark of *Boswellia serrata* is made into paste which is prescribed in case of snake-bites by the tribes of Hazaribagh district of Bihar.

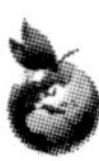

Bandicoot Berry

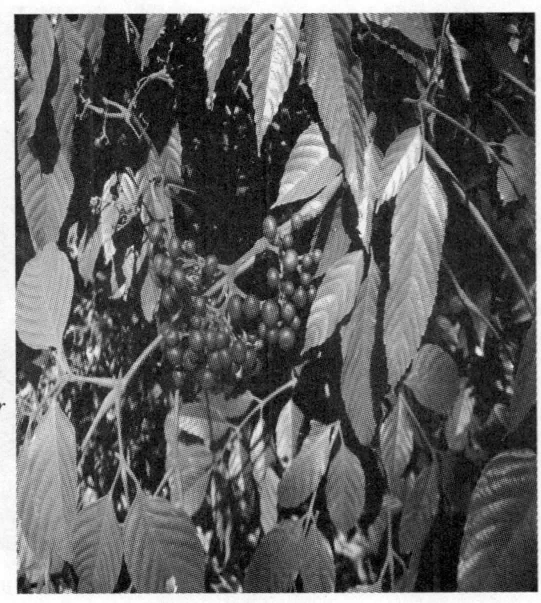

Botanical Name:
Leea indica

Family:
Leeaceae **(Leea family)**

Common Names:
Bandicoot Berry • Hindi: *Kukur jihwa* • Manipuri: *Koknal* • Marathi: *Karkani* • Tamil: Nalava, *Ottannalam* • Malayalam: *Nakku* • Telugu: *Amkador* • Kannada: *Gadhapatri* • Bengali: *Kurkur* • Assamese: *Ahina* • Sanskrit: *Chatri*

Description:
Bandicoot Berry is a shrub with straight branches. The leaves are double compound or triple compound, 90-120 cm long. The leaflets are extremely variable in size and shape. The flowers are greenish-white. The fruit is small. It is found in India to Indo-China, the Malay Peninsula, Java, Sumatra and Borneo.

Medicinal Uses:
A *decoction of the root* is given in *colic*, is *cooling* and *relieves thirst*. In Goa, the root is much used in *diarrhoeal* and *chronic dysentery*. The roasted leaves are applied to the head in *vertigo*. The *juice of the young leaves* is a *digestive*.

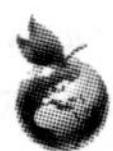

Garden Asparagus

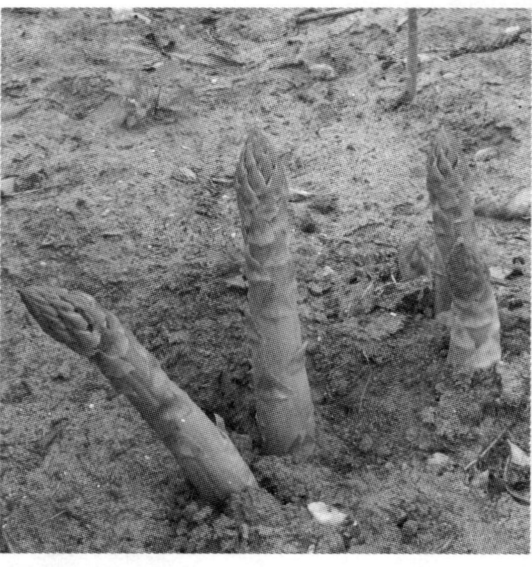

Botanical Name:
Asparagus officinalis

Family:
Liliaceae **(Lily family)**

Common Names:
Asparagus, Garden asparagus

Description:
Asparagus is believed to be native to the *east Mediterranean and the Middle-East.* It thrives along sandy riverbanks, shores of lakes and wet, salty coastal areas. It is very salt tolerant. Today it grows 'wild' across many of the areas around the world where it is grown for food. Asparagus grows into a tall upright bush. It's hard to say what the asparagus flower means. It's totally discrete. Hard to see, hard to study. Flowers are small, with two yellowish-green rings of petal-like tepals. Still, the asparagus flower is looked fro by the bees, the asparagus being honey-bearing. The leaves of the asparagus are even harder to define. They can't even remind of what usually defines a plant. The leaves barely have the shape of scales.

Medicinal Uses:
Vegetables eaten *raw or boiled*, the *asparagus has surprising medicinal properties.* The asparagus is indicated in some general illnesses like *asthenia, anoemia, rheumatism, diabetes* as well as *renal lithiasis. It is firstly a fortifier.* From the *asparagus offshoots, decoction, juice, syrup* and *tincture* are prepared. Very often, it is used is the *asparagus juice,* a preparation practically accessible to anyone.

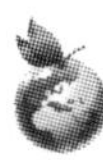

Satawari

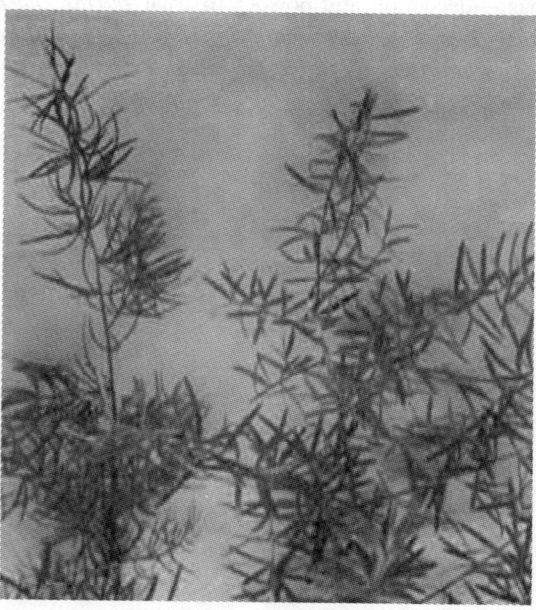

Botanical Name:

Asparagus racemosus

Family:

Liliaceae **(Lily family)**

Synonyms:

Asparagus volubilis

Common Names:

Satawari, Wild Asparagus • Hindi: *Satawari, Bojhidan, Shatavir* • Manipuri: *Nunggarei* • Marathi: *Satavari-mul, Asvel* • Tamil: *Sadavari, Tannir-muttan-kizhangu, Kilavari* • Malayalam *Chatavali, Satavali* • Telugu: *Challa-gaddalu, Challagadda, Ettavaludutige* • *Kannada: Aheruballi, Ashadhi, Halarru-makka*l • Bengali: *Satamuli, Satamul* • *Oriya*: Vari • *Urdu: Satawar, Shaqaqul misri* • Assamese: *Satomul* • *Sanskrit: Abhiru, Shatavari, Hiranyasringi* • Mizo: *Arkebawk*

Description:

Satawari is a woody climber growing to 1-2 m in height, with leaves like pine needles, small and uniform and the flowers white, in small spikes. It contains *adventitious root system* with *tuberous* roots. Stems are climbing, branched, up to 2 m; branches usually distinctly striate-ridged.

Leaves are just modified stems, called cladodes. Branches contain spines on them. Inflorescences develope after cladodes, axillary, each a many-flowered raceme or panicle about 1-4 cm.

Pedicel 1.5-3 mm, slender, articulate at middle. Flowers are white with a pink tinge, 2-3 mm, bell-shaped with 6 petals. Stamens equal, ca. 0.7 mm; anthers yellow and minute. Within India, it is found growing wild in tropical and sub-tropical parts of India including the Andamans; and ascending in the Himalayas up to an altitude of 1500 m. Flowering: October-November.

Medicinal Uses:

In *Ayurvedic medicine*, the *roots of Satavari* are used in the form of *juice*, paste, decoction and powder to treat *intrinsic haemorrhage, diarrhoea, piles, hoarseness of voice, cough, arthritis, poisoning, diseases of female genital tracts, erysipelas, fever,* as *aphrodisiac* and as a *rejuvinative.*

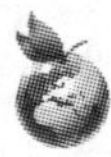

Kumarika

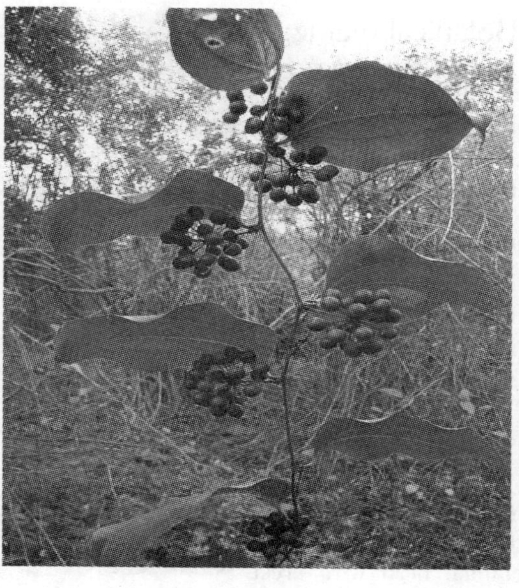

Botanical Name:
Smilax ovalifolia

Family:
Liliaceae **(Lily family)**

Synonyms:
Smilax macrophylla, Smilax zeylanica

Common Names:
Kumarika • Hindi: *Kumarika, Jangli aushbah, Bhitura* • Mizo: *Kaitha* • Marathi: *Ghotvel* • Tamil: *Ayadi, Malaittamarai, Tirunamappalai,* Kal *tamarai* • Malayalam: *Kaltamara, Karivilanti* • Telugu: *Kondadantena* • Kannada: *Kaadu hambu, Kaadu hambu thaavare* • Bengali: *Kumarika* • Oriya: *Mootrilata* • Sanskrit: *Vanamadhusnahi*

Description:
Kumarika is an armed or unarmed climber. Leaves leathery, shining, 7-15 x 4-11 cm, broadly ovate to elliptic, base rounded or shortly wedge-shaped; 3-5-nerved. Leaf stalk 1.5 cm long, base sheathing, with tendrils at the end. Flowers white, in dense umbels in leaf axils, 1-3 on a common peduncle. Bracts ovate. Perianth recurved in mature flowers, outer 3 segments, 4 mm long, oblong, inner narrower. Stamens about as long as the perianth. It is found from the Himalayan region in the north to Peninsular India. Flowering: January-April.

Medicinal Uses:
The *roots of* Kumarika are used for *veneral diseases.* It is also applied in *rheumatic swellings* and given in *urinary complaints* and *dysentery.*

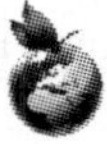

Flax

Botanical Name:
Linum usitatissimum

Family:
Linaceae **(Linseed family)**

Common Names:
Flax, Common flax, Flaxseed, Linseed • Hindi: *Alsi* • Tamil: *Ali* • Telugu: *Madanginja, Ullusulu* • Bengali: *Atasi* • Sanskrit: *Atasi*

Description:
Flax is a cool temperate annual herb with erect, slender stems, 80-120 cm tall. A cultivated plant in closely spaced field conditions it has little branching except at the apex.

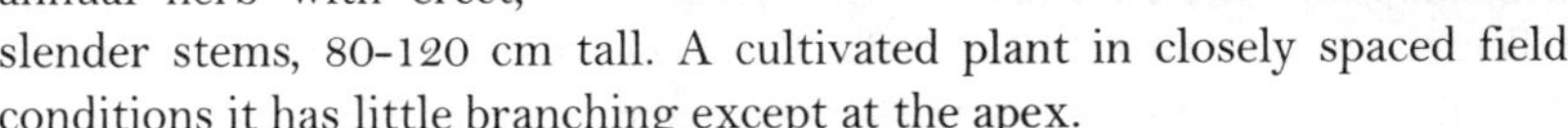

Leaves are alternate, lance-like and greyish-green with 3 veins. Flowers have five, pale blue petals in a cluster. The sepals are lance-like and nearly as long as the pointed fruit.

The fruit are spherical capsules. The seeds are oval, somewhat flattened, 4-6mm long and are pale to dark brown and shiny. Flax is native to the region extending from the eastern Mediterranean to India. It was extensively cultivated in ancient Egypt.

Flax is grown both for its seed and for its fibres. Interestingly, the species name *usitatissimum* means, most useful. Various parts of the plant have been used to make fabric, dye, paper, medicines, fishing nets and soap.

It is also grown as an ornamental plant in gardens, as flax is one of the few plant species capable of producing truly blue flowers (most "blue" flowers are really shades of purple), although not all flax varieties produce blue flowers. In Durga Puja, five flowers are offered to Goddess Durga, Red China Rose, Red Oleander, Lotus, Aparajita and Atasi (Flax).

Medicinal Uses:

In *Ayurveda*, Flax is used internally in *habitual constipation, functional disorders of the colon* resulting from the *misuse of laxatives* and *irritable colon*, as a *demulcent preparation in gastritis* and *enteritis.*

Externally, the powdered seeds or the press-cake are used as an *emollient*, in *poultices* for *boils, carbuncles* and other *skin afflictions.* It is used in *body lotions* to soothe the dry skin.

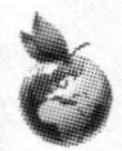

Nux Vomica

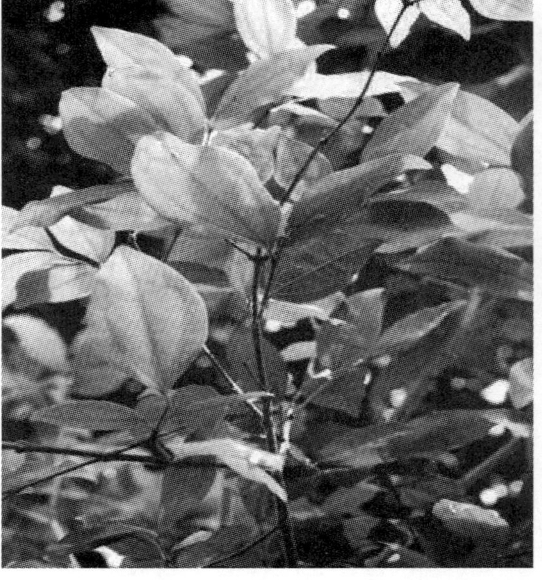

Botanical Name:

Strychnos nux-vomica

Family:

Loganiaceae **(Logania family)**

Common Names:

Nux Vomica, Poison Nut • Bengali: *Kuchila* • Hindi: *Bailewa, Chibbinge, Jahar, Kajra, Kucchla* • Kannada: *Hemmushti, Hemmusti, Ittangi* • Malayalam: *Chamram, Kanjiram, Kanni-rak-karu* • Marathi: *Kajra, Kuchala, Jharkhatchura* • Oriya: *Kuchla* • Sanskrit: *Kapilu, Chipita, Chutaka, Dirghapatra, Garadruma, Vishmushti* • Tamil: *Etti, Kagodi, Kalam, Kancirai* • Telugu: *Mucidi, Mushidi, Mushti* • Urdu: *Kuchla muddabir*

Description:

Nux Vomica is a medium-sized tree with a short, crooked, thick trunk. The wood is white hard, close grained and durable. Branches are irregular, covered with a smooth ash-coloured bark.

Young shoots are deep green, shiny. Oppostely arranged short stalked leaves are elliptic, shiny, smooth on both sides, about 4 inches long and 3 broad.

Flowers are small, greenish-white, funnel shaped, borne in small clusters at the end of branches They have a disagreeable smell. Fruit is about the size of a large apple with a smooth hard shell which when ripe is orange coloured, filled with a soft white jelly-like pulp containing five seeds.

The seeds are like flattened disks densely covered with closely appressed satiny hairs, radiating from the center of the flattened sides and giving to the seeds a characteristic sheen.

Medicinal Uses:

Nux Vomica is recommended for *upset stomach, vomiting, abdominal pains, constipation, intestinal irritation, hangovers, heartburn, insomnia, certain heart diseases, circulatory problems, eye diseases, depression, migraine headaches, nervous conditions, problems related to menopause* and *respiratory diseases* in the elderly. In *folk medicine,* it is used as *a healing tonic* and *appetite stimulant.*

Nux vomica is a common *homeopathic medicine* prescribed for *digestive problems, sensitivity to cold,* and *irritability.*

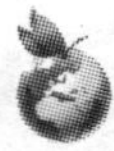

Blistering Ammannia

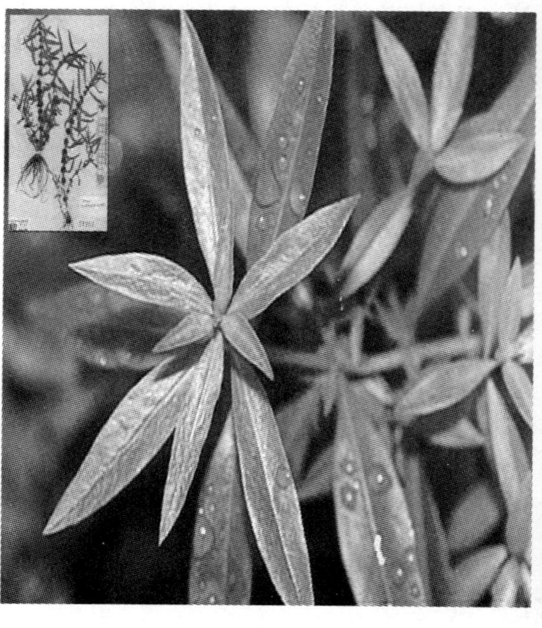

Botanical Name:
Ammannia baccifera

Family:
Lythraceae **(Crape Myrtle family)**

Synonyms:
Ammannia vescicatoria, Ammannia aegyptiaca

Common Names:
Blistering Ammannia, Acrid weed, Monarch redstem, Tooth cup • Hindi: *Aginbuti, Ban mirich, Dadmari, Jungli mehendi* • Marathi: *Aginbuti, Bharajambhula, Dadmari* • Tamil: *Kal-l-uruvi* • Malayalam: *Kallur vanchi, Nirumelneruppu* • Kannada: *Kaadugida* • Bengali: *Banmarich* • Konkani: *Dadmaria* • Sanskrit: *Agnigarbha, Brahmasoma, Kshetrabhusha, Kshetravashini, Mahasyama, Pasanabheda* • Nepali: *Ambar*

Description:
Blistering Ammannia is an erect, branched, smooth, slender, annual herb, found in open, damp, waste places. It is more or less purplish herb 10-50 cm in height, with somewhat 4-angled stems.

The leaves are narrow-oblong, oblance shaped, or narrowly elliptic, about 3.5 cm long - those on the branches very numerous, small, and 1-1.5 cm long – with narrowed base and pointed or somewhat rounded tip.

The flowers are small, about 1.2 mm long, greenish or purplish, and borne in dense clusters in leaf axils. The capsules are nearly spherical, depressed, about 1.2 mm in diameter, purple.

The seeds are black. The Common Names comes from the fact that the leaves are exceedingly acrid, irritant, and vesicant, and are being used by the village-folk to raise blisters, being applied to the skin for half an hour or a little longer.

Medicinal Uses:

The *leaves* or the *ashes of the plant, mixed with oil,* are applied to cure *herpetic eruptions.* The *fresh, bruised leaves* have been used in *skin diseases* as a *rubefacient* and as an *external remedy* for *ringworm and parasitic skin* infection.

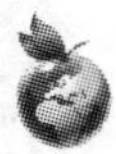

Common Crape Myrtle

Botanical Name:
Lagerstroemia indica

Family:
Lythraceae **(Crape Myrtle family)**

Common Names:
Crape myrtle • Hindi: Saoni • Marathi: *Dhayti* • Telugu: *Chinagoranta* • Tamil: *Pavalakkurinji*

Description:
Crape myrtle is the smaller version of *Lagerstroemia speciosa,* commonly known as Pride of India or Queen crape myrtle.

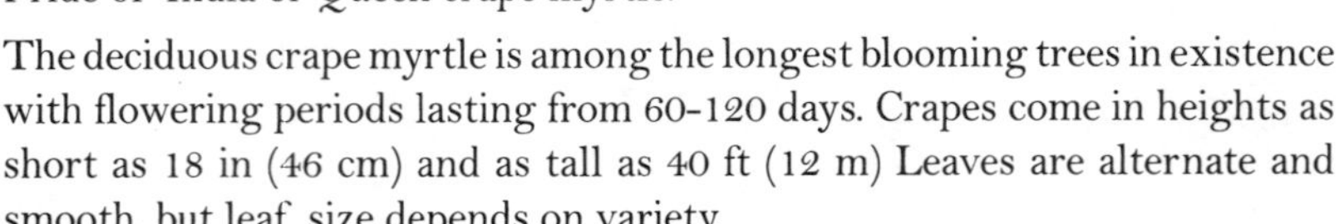

The deciduous crape myrtle is among the longest blooming trees in existence with flowering periods lasting from 60-120 days. Crapes come in heights as short as 18 in (46 cm) and as tall as 40 ft (12 m) Leaves are alternate and smooth, but leaf size depends on variety.

Flowers are borne in summer in big showy clusters and come in white and many shades of pink, purple, lavender and red.

Medicinal Uses:
Seeds are *narcotic.* In Manipur, *flowers* and *leaves* are used as *purgatives.* The bark is *stimulant* and *febrifuge* (fever removing) and *the roots* are *astringent* and used for gargle.

Queen Crape Myrtle

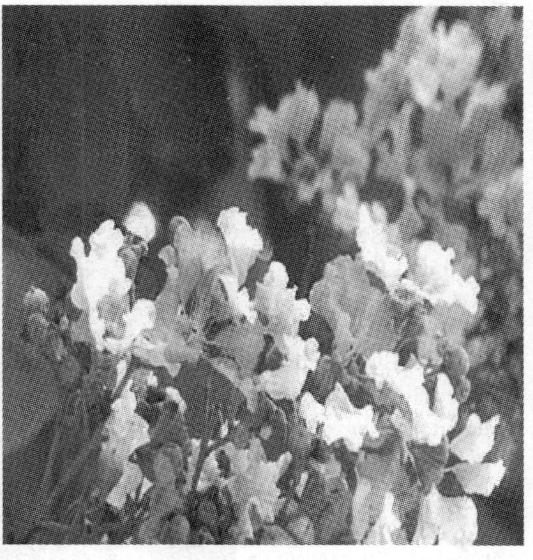

Botanical Name:

Lagerstroemia speciosa

Family:

Lythraceae **(Crape Myrtle family)**

Common Names:

Pride of India, Queen Crape Myrtle • Hindi: *Jarul* • Manipuri: *Jarol* • Tamil: *Kadali* • Marathi: *Taman*

Description:

This tropical flowering tree is one of the most outstanding summer bloomers. Lagerstroemia speciosa is a larger form of the more commonly grown L. indica (Crape myrtle.) It is called Queen Crape Myrtle because it's the Queen of the Crape Myrtles, dominating with grand size and larger, crinkled flowers. The name Crape myrtle is given to these tree/shrubs because of the flowers which look as if made from delicate crape paper. Lagerstroemia speciosa is a large tree growing up to 50' but it can be kept smaller by trimming. It stands on an attractive, spotted bark that often peels. This bark is commercially used and is a valuable timber. The large leaves are also appealing as they turn red right before they drop in the winter.

Medicinal Uses:

Seeds are *narcotic*, *bark and leaves* are *purgative*, *roots* are *astringent*, *stimulant* and *febrifuge* (fever removing) In Manipur, the fruit is used as *local application* for *apathy of the mouth*. *Decoction of dried leaves* is used in *diabetes*.

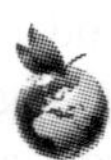

Fire Flame Bush

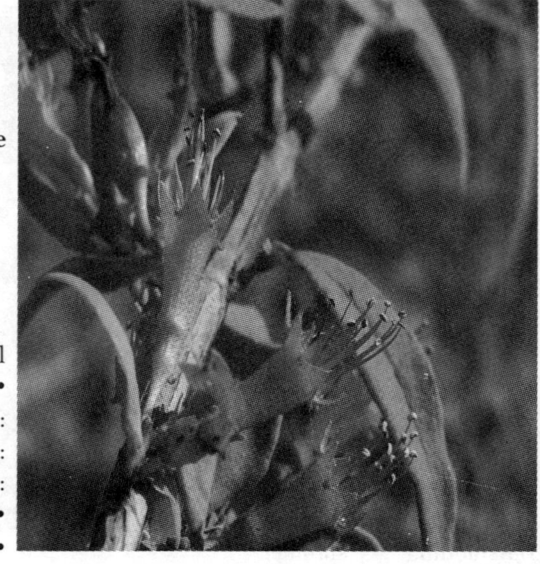

Botanical Name:
Woodfordia fruticosa

Family:
Lythraceae **(Crape Myrtle family)**

Synonyms:
Woodfordia floribunda

Common Names:
Fire Flame Bush, Red Bell Bush • Hindi: *Dhawai* • Marathi: *Dowari* • Tamil: *Velakkai* • Malayalam: *Tatiripuspi* • Telugu: *Jargi seringi, Godari* • Kannada: *Tamrapuspi* • Oriya: *Dhobo* • Konkani: *Dhauri* • Urdu: *Jetiko* • Gujarati: *Dhawani* • Sanskrit: *Parvati, Bahupuspika*

Description:
Fire Flame Bush is a spreading, leafy shrub, small in size but very conspicuous on dry, rocky hillsides from December to May, when the masses of little fiery bells give a bright touch of colour to the drab terrain. It is common in Sri Lanka, South Konkan and on the Ghats and ascends the Himalayas to 1500 m, but is rarer in South India.

It is a deciduous shrub, usually with a much-fluted stem. The grey bark is exceedingly thin and peels off in flakes. When in flower the bush appears twiggy and formless but entirely swathed in red.

This is because the small flowers grow singly or in groups all the way along the branches and side twigs, and it is at this time that the leaves fall. Each flower, borne on a tiny stem, is a slender tube, slightly curved, the greenish base of which is the sepal. Swelling slightly, the tube divides into narrow, pointed lobes and from within emerges a bunch of long stamens.

The whole length, including the stamens, is not more than 2 cm. The fruit is a small, oblong capsule, covered by the withered sepals. The narrow, pointed leaves grow straight from the branches, either opposite or in whorls of three.

They are harsh and dull, dark green in colour, but paler underneath. Sometimes they are dotted beneath with small, black glands. From the flowers, which contain much tannin, a red dye is obtained which is used to dye silks. The leaves also contain a large proportion of tannin and make the commonest tan in India.

Medicinal Uses:

This is a *drug* largely used in *native medicine.* This enters into the composition of many *preparations, decoctions, churnas* and *ghritas* for various diseases, but chiefly *dysentery* and *diarrhoea* by reason of its being highly *astringent.*

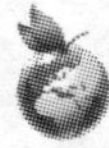

Madhavi Lata

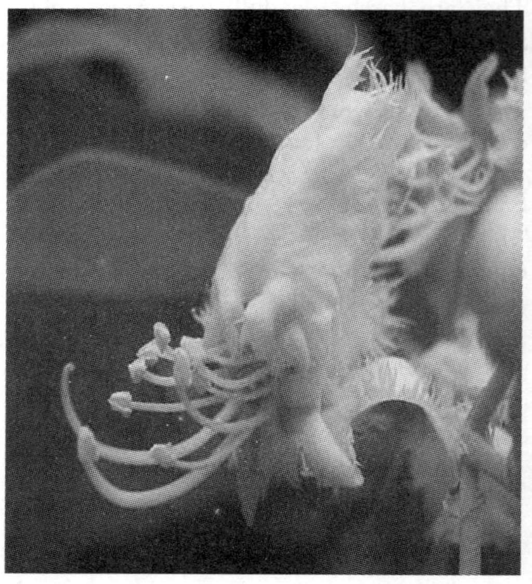

Botanical Name:

Hiptage benghalensis

Family:

Malpighiaceae **(Barbados cherry family)**

Common Names:

Hiptage, Helicopter Flower • Hindi: *Madhavi lata* • Manipuri: *Madhabi* • Kannada: *Madhvi* • Bengali: *Madhabilata* • Tamil: *Vasantakaala malligai*

Description:

Madhavi lata, native from India to the Philippines, is a vine like plant that is often cultivated in the tropics for its attractive and fragrant flowers. A woody climbing shrub with clusters of pink to white and yellow fragrant flowers and 3-winged, helicopter-like fruits. Flowers have very interesting shape and look like a decorative accessory, with fluffy-toothed edges. The fragrance is very strong and pleasant, resembles fruity perfume. Leaves are narrow and drooping. This plant can be trimmed as a bush, and can be crown in container, too. Used medicinally in India. Make sure to provide lots of light for profuse blooming. The genus name, *Hiptage*, is derived from the Greek hiptamai, which means "to fly" and refers its unique three-winged fruit known as "samara". The fruit is carried by wind because of its papery wings.

Medicinal Uses:

The *bark*, *leaves* and *flowers* are *aromatic*, *bitter*, *acrid*, *astringent*, *refrigerant*, *vulnerary*, *expectorant*, *cardio tonic*, *anti-inflammatory* and *insecticidal*. They are useful in *burning sensations*, *wounds*, *ulcers*, *cough*, and *asthma*.

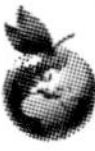

Barbados Cherry

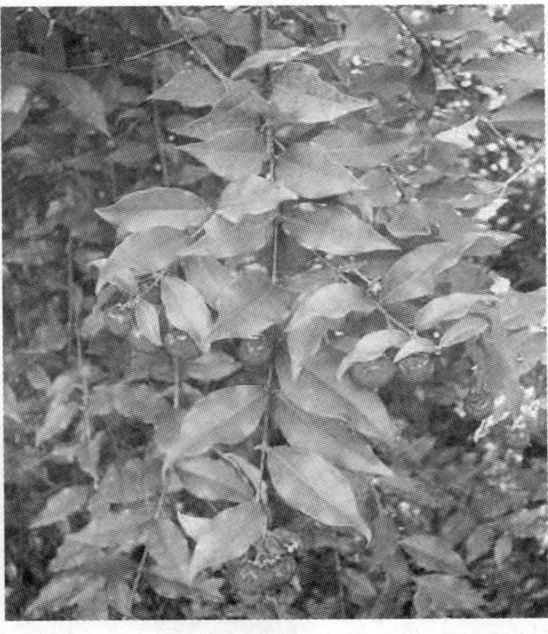

Botanical Name:

Malpighia glabra

Family:

Malpighiaceae **(Barbados cherry family)**

Common Names:

Barbados Cherry, Wild Crapemyrtle, Acerola

Description:

The Barbados cherry is a shrub or small tree that grows up to 15 feet tall with wide spread branches and evergreen oval leaves. The leaves are evergreen, simple, 0.5-15 cm long, with an entire, wavy margin. The flowers are solitary or in umbels of two to several together, each flower 1-2 cm diameter, with five pink or white petals. The fruit is a red, orange or purple drupe, containing 2-3 hard seeds. It is sweet and juicy, and very rich in vitamin C, up to 65 times that of an orange. Eaten fresh or as flavouring for drinks. Commonly used in parts of South America to *flavour ice creams, drinks* and *cocktails.*

Medicinal Uses:

In *Suriname's traditional medicine* the *leaves* are used against *dysentery* and *diarrhoea.* Also used for *liver ailments,* the *fruits* are used against *common cold.*

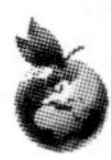

Indian Mallow

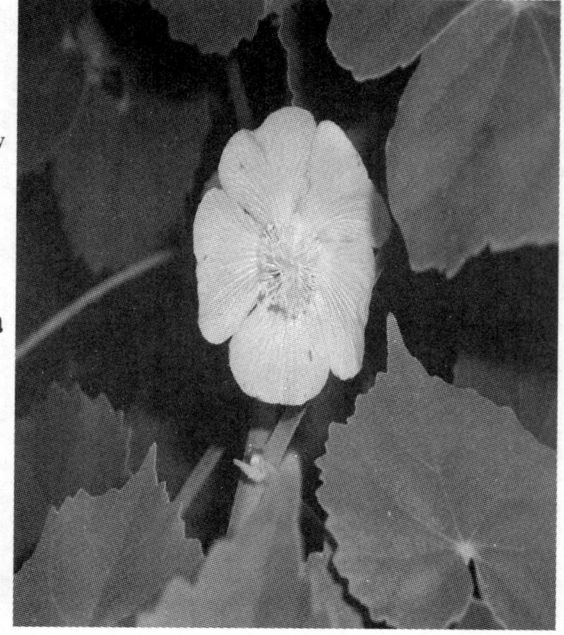

Botanical Name:
Abutilon indicum

Family:
Malvaceae **(Mallow family)**

Synonyms:
Sida indica

Common Names:
Indian Mallow, Country Mallow, Abutilon, Indian abutilon • Hindi: *Kanghi* • Marathi: *Petari* • Tamil: *Paniyaratutti* • Malayalam: *Velluram* • Telugu: *Tuturabenda* • Kannada: *Tutti* • Bengali: *Potari*

Description:
The Indian Mallow is an erect velvety-pubescent shrub with circular-ovate or heart-shaped leaves with coarsely crenate-serrate margins. The plant can reach up to 1-2 m.

The leaves are alternately arranged, and have long stalks and velvety, soft, pale hairs on them.

Orange-yellow flowers, 2-3 cm across, occur solitary in axils, on long stalks, 4-7 cm. Orange-yellow petals are triangular-obovate, 1 cm long or slightly more, staminal-tube hairy with stellate hairs.

The fruits are quite interesting, as - they are circular in shape, consisting of 11-20 radiating hairy carpels, brown when dry; each carpel flattened, somewhat boat shaped. Seeds are kidney-shaped.

The plant is a weed commonly found on disturbed land. Flowering: September-April.

Medicinal Uses:

The *extract of water-soaked dried seeds* is used as *a purgative.* Leaves are used as a *tonic* and *roots* are taken as *infusion in fever.*

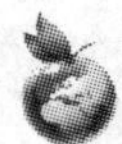

Bush Sorrel

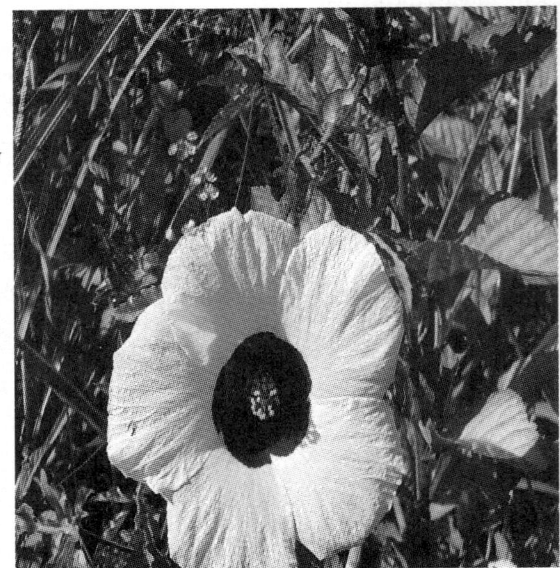

Botanical Name:
Hibiscus surattensis

Family:
Malvaceae **(Mallow family)**

Synonyms:
Furcaria surattensis

Common Names:
Bush Sorrel, Wild Sour, Bush Althea • Mizo: *Sehnap* • Tamil: *Kashlikirai, kattuppuliccai* • Malayalam: *Assam susor* • Telugu: *Mullugogu* • Kannada: *Mullu gogu*

Description:
Bush Sorrel is a weak-stemmed, prostrate or climbing plant covered with soft hairs and scattered prickles. The leaves are rounded, up to 10 X 10 cm, and deeply and palmately 3- to 5-lobed, the lobes being toothed.

The flowers are yellow, with a dark center, and occur singly in leaf axils. Petals are obovate, up to 6 cm long and 4 cm wide. This flower can be easily identified by its unique false sepals, which are 8-10 in number.

The false sepals (actually bracts) are forked into a spoon-shaped outer part, and a narrow linear inner part. But for this feature, the plant can be confused with Deccan Hemp.

The capsules are hairy and ovoid. The seeds are downy. Bush Sorrel is found throughout the tropical world. Its leaves are commonly used as pot-herb in many parts of Africa and Asia. Flowering: September-March.

Medicinal Uses:

In Senegal, the *plant* is used as an *emollient.* Watt and Breyer-Brandwijk report that the Zulus use a *lotion of the leaf* and *stem for the treatment of penile irritation* of any sort, including *venereal sores* and *urethritis.*

It is sometimes applied as an *ointment* for the same purposes. An *infusion* is also used as an *injection* into the *urethra* and the *vagina* for *gonorrhoea* and other *inflammations.*

Fragrant Swamp Mallow

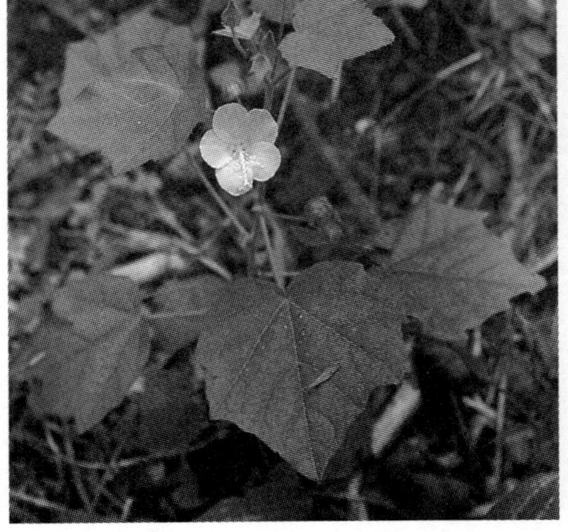

Botanical Name:
Pavonia odorata

Family:
Malvaceae (**Mallow family**)

Common Names:
Fragrant Swamp Mallow, Pavonia, Fragrant Pavonia • Hindi: *Sugandhabala* • Marathi: *Sugandhabala, Kalavala* • Tamil: *Peramutti, Avibattam* • Malayalam: *Iruveli, Kuruntotti* • Telugu: *Chittibenda, Ettakuti* • Kannada: *Balarakshi gida* • Gujarati: *Kalowalo* • Sanskrit: *Udichya, Varinamaka, Hribera, Valaka*

Description:
Fragrant Swamp Mallow is an erect perennial herb, covered with sticky hairs. Leaves are heart-shaped-ovate, 3-5 angled or 3-5 lobed, 4-6 cm long, 5-7 cm broad. Flowers arise singly in leaf axils, or fascicled at the end of branches. Bracts are 10-12 in number, linear, and sepals are 5. Flowers are pink, twice longer than the sepal cup. Fruit is spherical and mericarps smooth, wingless. Fragrant Swamp Mallow is found in India, Pakistan, Burma, Sri Lanka and East Tropical Africa.

Medicinal Uses:
The *plant* is used in *Ayurvedic medicine.* A *powder* is obtained by grinding the dried roots of Fragrant Swamp Mallow. This powder is used for *skin conditioning* and *soothing.*

Indian Tulip Tree

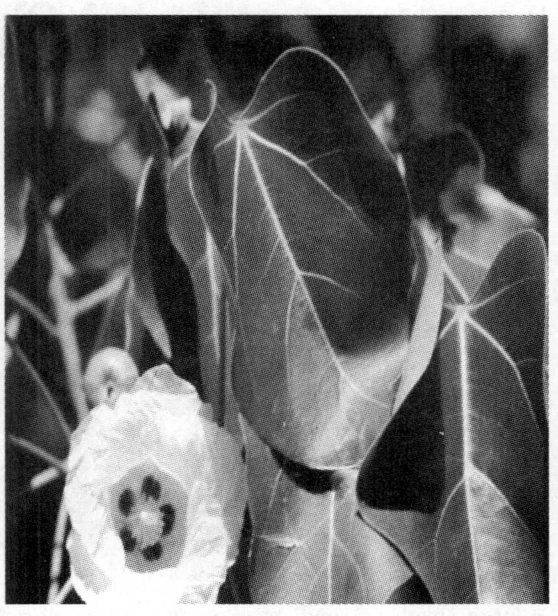

Botanical Name:
Thespesia populnea

Family:
Malvaceae **(Mallow family)**

Common Names:
Indian tulip tree, Aden apple, Portia tree • Hindi: *Paras pipal* • Malayalam: *Puvarasu* • Bengali: *Palaspipal* • Tamil: *Puvarasu*

Description:
This is a good tree for small gardens or patios. Its name Thespesia means "divinely decreed" and was given by Daniel Solander who saw it in Tahiti as a member of Captain Cook's ship. Indian tulip tree is an evergreen bushy tree. It grows to 40 ft or more with a spread of 10–20 ft. It has heart-shaped leaves and cup-shaped yellow flowers that are produced intermittently throughout the year in warm climates. Each flower has a maroon eye that ages to purple. The flowers are followed by apple-shaped fruit.

Medicinal Uses:
Ground up bark is used to treat *skin diseases* (India), *dysentery* and *haemorrhoids* (Mauritius). *Leaves* are applied to *inflamed and swollen joints* (South India). When cut, the *young fruit* secretes a *yellow sticky* sap used to treat *ringworm* and other *skin diseases* (South India). *Roots* are used as a *tonic.* There is some modern investigation of the *plant's effects on high blood pressure.*

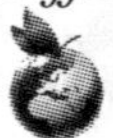

Ironwood Tree

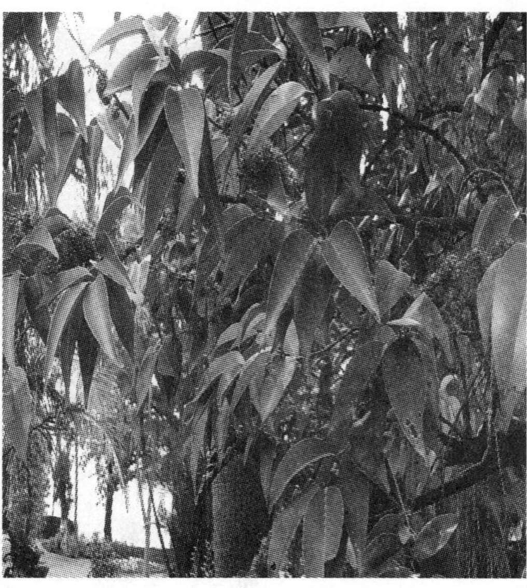

Botanical Name:
Memecylon umbellatum

Family:
Melastomataceae
(Melastome family)

Synonyms:
Memecylon edule

Common Names:
Delek air tree, Ironwood tree • Hindi: *Anjan, Kaya* • Marathi: *Anjan* • Telugu: *Mandi, Lakhonde* • Malayalam: *Kanjavu* • Oriya: *Neymaru*

Description
A large shrub or small tree, up to 8-14m tall with amazing bright blue flowers that look almost unreal. Delek air produces showy clusters of tiny purple flowers, about 1cm each. The trees bloom once or twice a year, and are then indeed a beautiful sight. As the flower petals are shed, the sand and rocks below are dusted in mauve. The fruits are small (about 1cm) and are green, turning red then black as they ripen. The tree has a thin bark, so it is sometimes also called 'Nipis kulit' or 'thin-skinned' in Malay. Delek air belongs to the same family as the more familiar Singapore Rhododendron (Melastoma malabathricum). This tree is not only beautiful, but also useful. It provides hard timber used for building houses and boats. *A yellow dye can be extracted from the leaves and the bark is used to treat bruises.*

Medicinal Uses:
The *leaves* are used in the *treatment of gonorrhoea*, or when mixed with several other ingredients, they make *good fomentations for external use.*

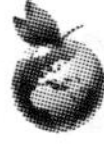

Pithraj Tree

Botanical Name:
Aphanamixis polystachya

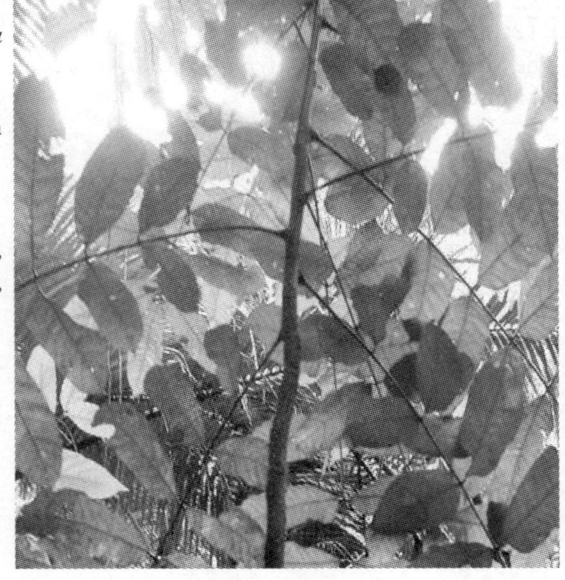

Family:
Meliaceae **(Neem family)**

Synonyms:
Aglaia polystachya, Amoora rohituka, Andersonia rohituka

Common Names:
Pithraj Tree
• Hindi: *Harin-hara, Harinkhana* • Manipuri: *Heirangkhoi* • Marathi: *Raktharohida* • Tamil: *Malampuluvan, Sem, Semmaram* • Malayalam: *Chemmaram, Sem* • Telugu: *Chevamanu, Rohitaka* • Kannada: *Mukhyamuttage, Mullumuttaga, Mulluhitthalu, Roheethaka* • Bengali: *Tiktaraj* • *Kuki: Sahala* • Khasi: *Dieng rata* • *Rongmei: Agan* • Assamese: *Hakhori bakhori* • Sanskrit: *Anavallabha, Ksharayogya, Lakshmi, Lakshmivana, Lohita*

Description:
The Pithraj Tree is a deciduous tree native to India, growing to 20-30 m tall. Leaves are odd- or even- pinnate, 30-60 cm long, with 9-21 leaflets. Leaflets are oblong-elliptic, elliptic, or ovate, 17-26 × 4-10 cm with basal pair smallest, leathery when mature, with visible transparent tiny spots under sunlight. Base of the leaflets is oblique, margin entire.

Flower clusters occur in leaf axils, less than a foot long. Flowers are 6-7 mm in diameter, with three bracteoles.

Flowers have five nearly circular sepals, 1-1.5 mm across. Petals are 3-7 mm in diameter, concave. Staminal tube is spherical, smooth. Anthers are 5 or 6, and oblong.

Capsule is sort of ovoid, 2-2.5 × 2.5-3 cm, orangish when mature. Seeds are greyish brown. Flowering: May-September.

Medicinal Uses:

The *bark* is used in *spleen, liver diseases, tumour and abdominal complaints.* Seed-oil is used in *rheumatism.*

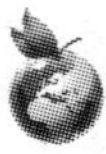

Ranabili

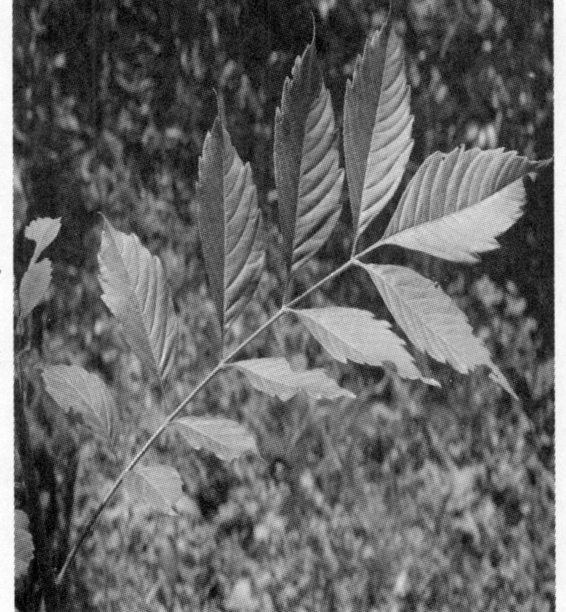

Botanical Name:

Cipadessa baccifera

Family:

Meliaceae **(Neem family)**

Synonyms:

Melia baccifera, Cipadessa fruticosa

Common Names:

Ranabili • Hindi: *Nalbila* • Marathi: *Ranabili, Gudmai* • Tamil: *Puilipan cheddi* • Malayalam: *Kaipanarangi*, Potti, *Pulippanchedi* • Kannada: *Narsullu*, Chitunde, *Karbe* • Urdu: *Ranabili*

Description:

Ranabili is a shrub 1-4 m tall, with coarse bark. Young branches are grayish brown, ribbed, and covered with yellow velvety hairs and sparse grayish white lenticels.

Leaves are compound, 8-30 cm long, with leaf-stalk and spine either hairless or yellow velvety. Leaflets are usually 9-13, opposite, ovate to ovoid-oblong, 3.5-10 × 1.5-5 cm.

Flowers are born in clusters 8-15 cm long. Flowers are white, 3-4 mm in diameter. Flower stalks are 1-1.5 mm long. Sepal cup is short, yellow velvety outside. Sepals are broadly triangular.

Petals are white or yellow, linear to oblong-elliptic, 2-3.5 mm, outside covered with sparse appressed velvety hairs. Stamens are shorter than petals, with hairy filaments. Fruit is purple to black when mature, round, 4–5 mm in diameter. Flowering: April-October.

Medicinal Uses:

The juice of the root is given in cases of *indigestion.* It is also used in treating *cough and cold.*

A paste of the bark is pressed against the teeth for about 15 minutes to *relieve bleeding* and *swelling of gums.*

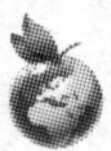

Persian Lilac

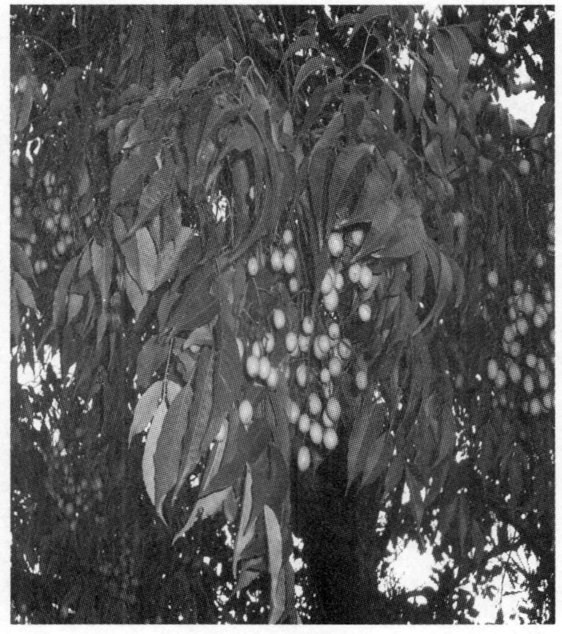

Botanical name:
Melia azedarach

Family:
Meliaceae **(Mahogany family)**

Synonyms:
Melia azedarach var. japonica, Melia toosendan

Common Names:
Chinaberry tree, Persian lilac, Pride of India, Bead tree, Lilac tree • Hindi: *Bakain* • Manipuri: *Seizrak* • Marathi: *Bakan-nimb* • Bengali: *Bakarjam* • Tamil: *Kattu vembhu*

Description:
The Persian lilac tree is frequently confused with Neem. However, the structure of the leaves and the colour of the flowers, white in Neem and lilac in Persian lilac, are sufficient to distinguish between the two.

A large evergreen tree native to India, growing wild in the sub-Himalayan region. In India, Muslims are credited with the spread of the tree. The bark is reddish brown, becoming fissured on mature trees.

The deciduous leaves are bipinnate (twice feather-like) and 1-2 ft long. The individual leaflets, each about 2 in long and less than half as wide, are pointed at the tips and have toothed edges.

In spring and early summer, Persian lilac produces masses of purplish, fragrant, star shaped flowers, each about 3/4 in in diameter, that arch or droop in 8 in panicles. They are followed by clusters of spherical, yellow fruits about 3/4 in in diameter that persist on the trees even after the leaves have fallen.

All parts of Persian lilac tree are poisonous. Eating as few as 6 berries can result in death. Birds that eat too many seeds have been known to become paralyzed.

Medicinal Uses:

The *bark and fruit extract* is used to kill *parasitic roundworms.* In Manipur, *leaves and flowers* are used as *poultice in nervous headaches.*

Leaves, bark and *fruits* are *insect repellant. Seed-oil* is used *in rheumatism and* wood-extract is used in *asthma.*

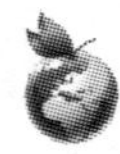

Gulbel

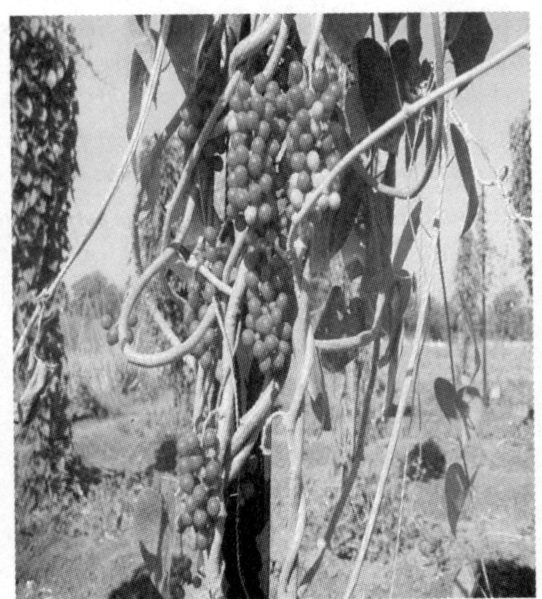

Botanical Name:

Tinospora cordifolia

Family:

Menispermaceae
(Moonseed family)

Common Names:

Gulbel, Indian Tinospora • Hindi: *Giloy, Gulancha, Gulbel* • Manipuri: *Ningthou khongli* • Marathi: *Gulvel* • Tamil: *Kunali* • Telugu: *Manapala* • Kannada: *Madhuparni* • Bengali: *Nimgilo* • Konkani: *Amritvel* • Assamese: *Hoguni*-lot • Sanskrit: *Guruchi*

Description:

Gulbel is a native plant from India, also known to be found in Far East, primarily in rainforests.

The plant is climbing shrub with heart-shaped leaves. It has stems about 6 cm in diameter, with light grey, papery bark. The leaves are 7.5-14 cm long, 9-17 cm broad, broadly ovate or orbicular, deeply heart shaped at the base. Tiny greenish yellow flowers occur in racemes 7-14 cm long.

Flowers have 3+3 sepals in 2 layers, the outer ones are small, the inner large. Six stamens prominently protrude out.

The plant flowers during the summer and fruits during the winter. Gulbel prefers acid, neutral or basic alkaline soil.

It can grow in semi-shade or no shade. Requiring moist soil. Gulbel grows easily without chemical fertilizers, and use of pesticides.

Medicinal Uses:

The herb has a long history in use by practitioners of *Ayurved.* Known by its practitioners to treat *convalescence from severe illness, arthritis* (or joint *diseases*), *liver diseases, eye diseases, urinary problems, anaemia, cancer, diarrhoea,* and *diabetes.* Also, it helps *remove toxins from the body.*

The plant is cultivated by stem cutting in the month of May-June and used in *Tibetan medicine.* The herb is known to have a sweet, bitter and *acid taste.*

Extracted from the *stem and root is a nutrient starch* used to treat *chronic diarrhoea* and *dysentery.* According to a legend, the herb is known locally as *giloya* or 'heavenly elixir', which means, 'Kept the angels eternally young'.

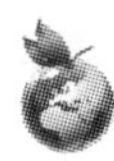

Shikakai

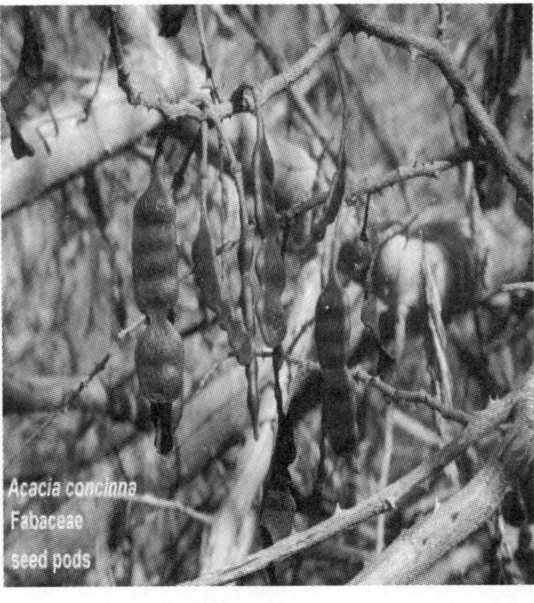

Botanical Name:

Acacia concinna

Family:

Mimosaceae **(Touch-me-not family)**

Synonyms:

Acacia hooperiana, Acacia sinuata, Mimosa concinna

Common Names:

Shikakai, Soap-pod • Hindi: *Kochi, Reetha, Shikakai* • Marathi: Reetha • Tamil: *Shika, Sheekay,* Chikaikkai • Malayalam: *Cheeyakayi, Chinik-kaya, Shikai, Cheenikka* • Telugu: *Cheekaya, Chikaya, Gogu* • Kannada: *Sheegae, Shige kayi, Sigeballi* • Oriya: *Vimala* • Urdu: *Shikakai* • Assamese: *Amsikira, Kachuai, Pasoi tenga, Suse lewa* • Sanskrit: *Bahuphenarasa, Bhuriphena, Charmakansa, Charmakasa, Phenila*

Description:

Shikakai is a climbing, most well-known for the natural shampoo derived from its fruit. Thorny branches have brown smooth stripes - thorns are short, broad-based, flattened.

Leaves with caducous stipules not thorn-like. Leaf stalks are 1-1.5 cm long with a prominent gland about the middle. Leaves are double-pinnate, with 5-7 pairs of pinnae, the primary rachis being thorny, velvety.

Each pinnae has 12-18 pairs of leaflets, which are oblong-lanceshaped, 3-10 mm long, pointed, obliquely rounded at base.

Inflorescences is a cluster of 2 or 3 stalked rounded flower-heads in axils of upper reduced leaves, appearing paniculate. Stalk carrying the cluster is 1-2.5 cm long, velvety.

Flower-heads about 1 cm in diameter when mature. Flowers are pink, without or with reduced subtending bracts. Pods are thick, somewhat flattened, stalked, 8 cm long, 1.5-1.8 cm wide.

Medicinal Uses:

Shikakai is a commonly used *herb* that has many *remedial qualities.* It is popularly referred as *'fruit for the hair'* as it has a naturally *mild pH,* that gently cleans the hair without stripping it of *natural oils.*

Shikakai is used to *control dandruff, promoting hair growth* and *strengthening hair roots.* Its leaves are used in *malarial fever,* and *decoction of the pods* are used to *relieve biliousness* and *acts as a purgative.*

An *ointment,* prepared from the ground pods, is good for *skin diseases.*

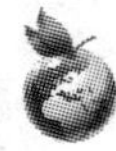

Eucalyptus

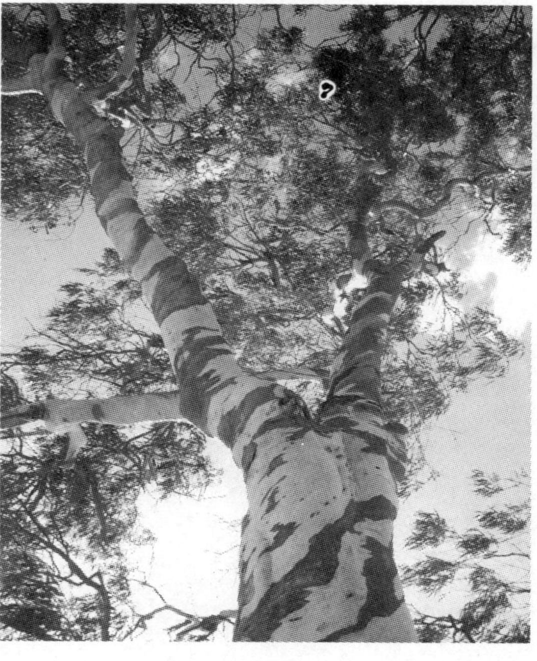

Botanical Name:
Eucalyptus spp.

Family:
Myrtaceae **(Myrtle Family)**

Common Names:
Eucalyptus • Hindi: *Safeda* • Manipuri: *Nasik*

Description:
Eucalyptus is a diverse genus of trees (rarely shrubs), the members of which dominate the tree flora of Australia.

All eucalypts are evergreen, although some species have deciduous bark. On warm days vapourised eucalyptus oil rises above the bush to create the characteristic distant blue haze of the Australian landscape.

Eucalyptus oil is highly flammable (trees have been known to explode) and bush fires can travel easily through the oil-rich air of the tree crowns. Eucalypts exhibit leaf dimorphism.

When young, the leaves are opposite and often roundish and occasionally without petiole. When several years old, the leaves become quite slender and with long petiole.

Eucalyptus flowers typically vary from white, cream, pink, yellow, or red depending upon the species. The flower petals and stamens are fused into a cap called an operculum — as the flower opens the cap is shed.

The flowers appear as a fuzzy, cream-yellow ball of stamens. After flowering, hard, woody seed pods develop and are often key to identifying the plant species. Typically, these seed heads remain on the tree until released by fire or the plant's death.

Medicinal Uses:

Eucalyptus oil has medicinal properties - the well-known, *Vicks vapo-rub* is made out of *eucalyptus oil.*

Traditionally, *eucalyptus oil* is known to be a *good medicine* for *relieving nasal congestion and cold.*

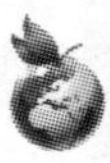

Malay Apple

Botanical Name:
Syzygium malaccense

Family:
Myrtaceae
(Bottlebrush family)

Synonyms:
Eugenia malaccensis, Jambosa malaccensis

Common Names:
Malay Apple, Mountain Apple, Rose Apple • Hindi: *Malay jamun* • Bengali: *Malaka jamrul* • Assamese: *Pani-jamuk*

Description:
Malay Apple is a native fruit of Malaysia, but has been introduced in many tropical countries, including India. It is a medium sized tree, growing up to 60 ft tall.

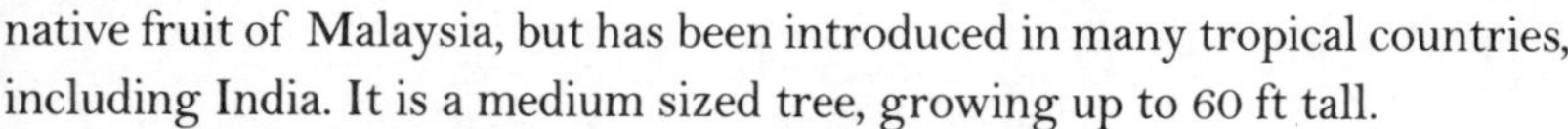

The evergreen leaves are opposite, soft leathery and dark green: the flowers are purplish - red and form a carpet after falling under the tree. The fruit is oblong to pear shaped with a dark red skin and white flesh; sometimes it is seedless.

The fruit is oblong-shaped and dark red in colour, although some varieties have white or pink skin. The flesh is white and surrounds a large seed.

The flesh makes a jam prepared by stewing with brown sugar and ginger. The trunk of the Mountain Apple tree was used by the people of old Hawaii to build beams for their hale, house and for fashioning bowls and poi-boards.

A reddish brown dye for making patterns on tapa bark cloth, was processed from the bark and the root.

Medicinal Uses:

A *decoction of the bark* is used against *vaginal infections*, while the root is used to treat itching.

The *root* is also effective against *dysentery* and as a *diuretic*. In Brazil, the plant is also used as a *remedy for diabetes* and *constipation*.

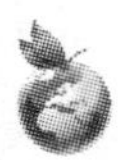

Red Spiderling

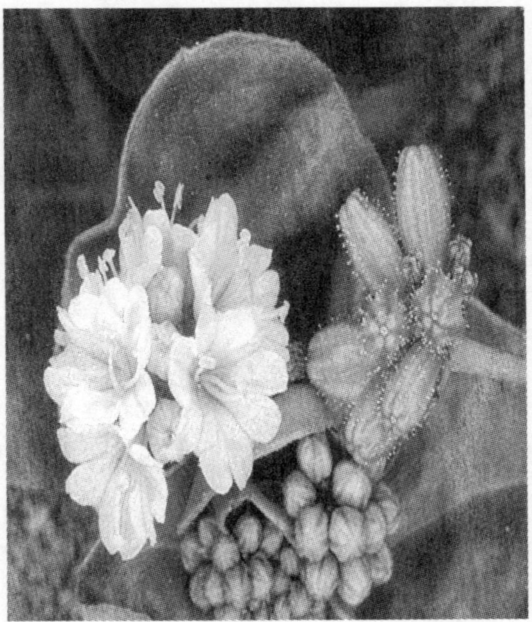

Botanical Name:
Boerhavia diffusa

Family:
Nyctaginaceae
(Bougainvillea family)

Synonyms:
Boerhavia repens,
Boerhavia coccinea

Common Names:
Red hogweed, Tar Vine, Red Spiderling, Wineflower • Hindi: *Punarnava, Satha* • Kannada: *Adakaputtana gida*

Description:
Red Spiderling is a prostrate herb with very diffuse inflorescences. It is a weed found throughout India. Inflorescences occur at the end of branches, are forked about 3-6 times, occasionally with sticky internodal bands.

Branches are divergent, terminating in compact subumbellate or capitate, 2-5-flowered clusters. Flowers have stalk shorter than 0.5 mm. Bract at base of the flower tube quickly deciduous, lancelike, 0.8-1 mm.

Flowers are purplish red to reddish pink or nearly white, bell-shaped beyond the constriction, 1-1.5 mm. Stamens 2-3, are inside the flower or barely protruding out.

Tender young leaves and shoots are cooked and used as a vegetable.

Medicinal Uses:

Popular in *Ayurveda,* this *herb* is known for *its anti-inflammatory* and *analgesic properties.*

The *roots* of Boerhavia diffusa, commonly known as 'Punarnava', are used by a large *number of tribes in India* for the treatment of various *hepatic disorders* and for *internal inflammation.*

Anodectal data has also reported effectiveness of Boerhavia diffusa in cases of *oedema* and *ascites* resulting from *early cirrhosis of the liver* and *chronic peritonitis.*

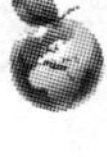

Yellow Jasmine

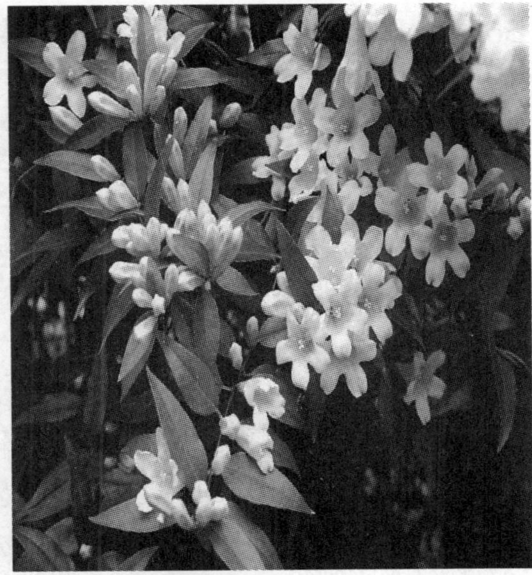

Botanical Name:
Jasminum humile

Family:
Oleaceae **(Jasmine family)**

Synonyms:
Jasminum wallichianum, Jasminum revolutum, Jasminum pubigerum

Common Names:
Yellow Jasmine, Italian Jasmine • Hindi: *Peeli chameli* • Nepali: *Masino Jaai*

Description:
Yellow Jasmine is a small erect much-branched shrub, growing to 1 m or more tall, commonly found in the Himalayan region. It has green, angular branches. Leaves are pinnate with 3-7 ovate to lancelike leathery leaflets. The last leaflet is somewhat larger. Inflorescences are lax clusters of yellow tubular flowers at the end of branches. Flowers have a slender tube, 1-2 cm long, with 5 rounded spreading petals, about 6 mm. Sepal tube is cup shaped, only 3 mm in size, with tiny triangular sepals. Fruit is black berry, 8 mm in size, with crimson juice. Flowering: April-June.

Medicinal Uses:
The *flowers* are *astringent and a tonic for the heart and bowels.* A *paste made from the flowers* is considered effective in the treatment of *intestinal problems.* The *juice of the roots* is used in *the treatment of ringworm.* The *milky juice of the plant* is used for destroying *the unhealthy lining walls of chronic sinuses and fistulas.*

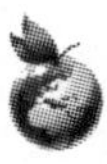

Weaver`s Beam Tree

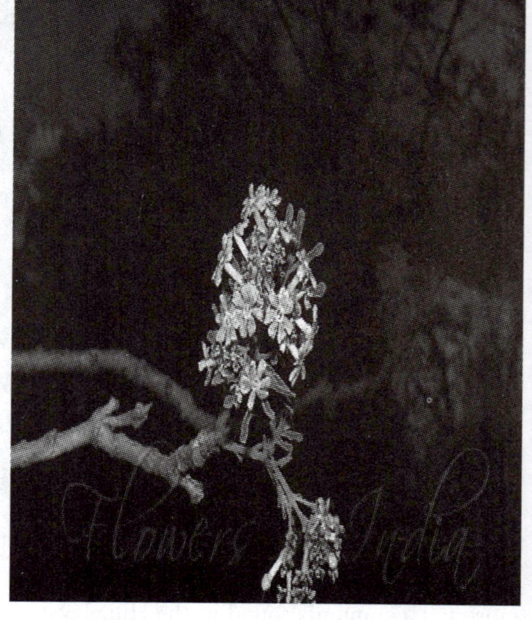

Botanical Name:

Schrebera swietenioides

Family:

Oleaceae **(Jasmine family)**

Common Names:

Weaver's Beam Tree • Hindi: *Banpalas, Mokhdi, Mokha* • Kannada: *Bula, gante, Mogalingamara* •Malayalam: Maggamaram, Malamplasu, Muskkakavrksam • Marathi: *Mokha, Mokadi, Nakti* • Oriya: *Mokka* • *Sanskrit: Ghantapatali, Golidha, Kastapatola* • Tamil: *Kattupparutticceti, Mogalingam, Makalinkam* • Telugu: *Bullakaya, Magalinga, Tondamukkudi*

Description:

Weaver's Beam Tree is a moderate sized deciduous tree, growing up to 20 m tall, with thick grey bark. Leaves are pinnate, with 3-4 pairs of opposite leaflets, and a terminal one.

Leaflets are ovate, entire, unequal-sided, petioles thickened at the insertion of leaflets. Flowers are yellowish white, variegated with brown, in terminal trichotomous, corymb-like, compound clusters. Flowers are fragrant at night.

Flower tube is funnel- shaped, 8-12 mm long. Petals are 5-7, widely spreading, wedge-shaped, blunt, with brown glandular raised dots on the upper side.

Capsule is the size of a hen's egg, pear-shaped, woody, hard, scabrous, 2-celled, seeds 4 in each cell, pendulous, irregularly oval, compressed, produced into a long membranous wing.

The wood is used by weavers to make the beam of the looms. Flowering: February-April.

Medicinal Uses:

The *roots, bark* and *leaves* are *bitter, acrid, appetising, digestive, thermogenic, stomachic, depurative, constipating urinary astringent* and *anthelmintic.* The fruits are reported to be useful in curing *hydrocele.*

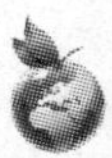

River Beauty

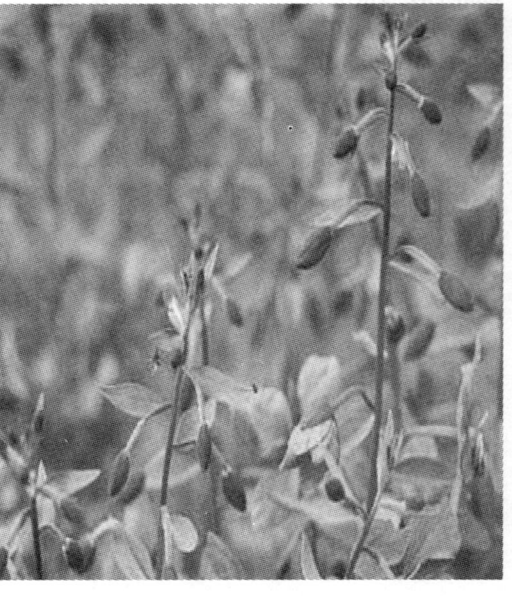

Botanical Name:
Epilobium latifolium

Family:
Onagraceae **(Evening primrose family)**

Common Names:
River Beauty, Dwarf Fireweed

Description:
A deciduous perennial that grows to 1.0 meters (3.3 feet) high by 0.5 meters (1.65 feet) wide and prefers many types of soil with a pH ranging from acid to alkaline and partial to full sun with moderate moisture. This plant withstands frost and has hermaphrodite flowers. Leaves narrow-elliptic, hairy beneath. Four petalled purplish pink flowers are 5 cm across, in leafy spike-like terminal clusters. Found in the Himalayas and the Uttarakhand hill stations. River gravels, margins of streams and damp slopes.

Medicinal Uses:
The entire plant is used in *Tibetan medicine.* It is said to have a *bitter taste* and a *cooling potency. Analgesic, antidote, anti-inflammatory, antipruritic, antirheumatic* and *febrifuge*, it is used in the treatment of *fevers and inflammations*, plus for *itching pimples.*

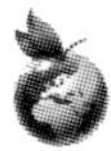

Evening Primrose

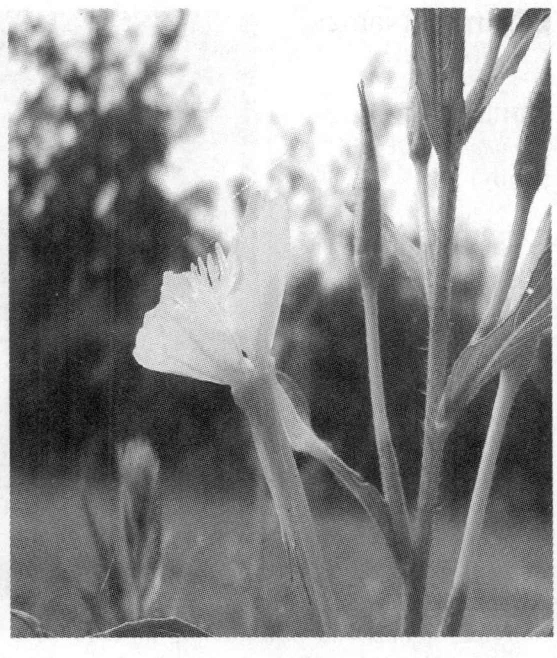

Botanical Name:
Oenothera biennis

Family:
Onagraceae **(Evening primrose family)**

Common Names:
Evening Primrose, Common Evening Primrose

Description:
Evening primrose, the beautiful yellow flower, gets its name from the fact that it remains partially close in the day, and opens up suddenly in the evening. Oenothera family is highly variable, and hence difficult to identify. The plant has an upright stem with leaves that are 10-20 cm long, slightly toothed and lance like. Flowers are large, yellow, 2.5-5 cm wide, with four petals. A cross-shaped stigma protrudes out of the flower cup.

Medicinal Uses:
The plant contains *an astringent mucilage* that modern herbalists use in *cough remedies.* Externally, the plant has been used to *treat sores* and *various skin conditions.* Published studies indicate that the oil might be useful in *treating atopic eczema* or *eczema* caused by *allergies.*

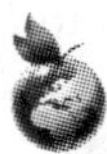

Crested Coelogyne

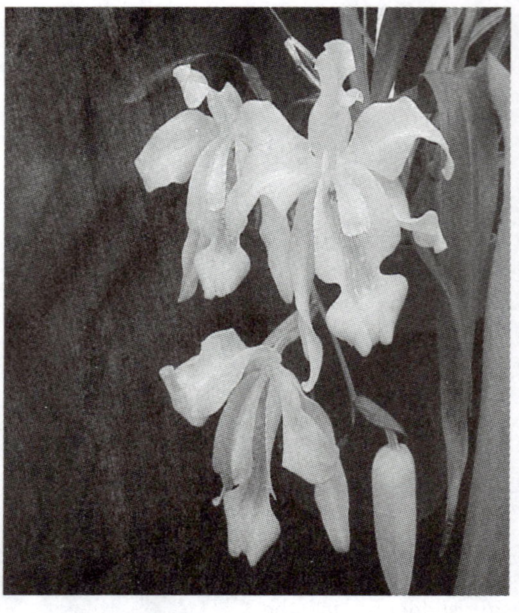

Botanical Name:

Coelogyne cristata

Family:

Orchidaceae **(Orchid family)**

Common Names:

Crested Coelogyne • Hindi: *Gondya* • Nepali: *Chandi gabha*

Description:

Crested Coelogyne is a very common orchid found growing on forest trees in the Himalayas, from Uttarakhand to Sikkim, at altitudes of 1000-2000 m. Joseph Hooker, who collected orchids and other plants in 1848-1850, recorded that *"On the ascent from Darjeeling the straight shafts of many of the timber trees are literally clothed with a continuous garment of white-flowered coelogynes, which bloom in a profuse manner, whitening their trunks like snow"*. Flowers are white, in hanging clusters, with a white lip with four yellow ridges at the base between the lateral lobes, and with two broad crenulate yellow plates on the mid-lobe. Flowers are 5-9 cm across, borne in 3-10 flowered clusters 15-20 cm long. Sepals and petals are 4-5 cm long, oblong blunt with wavy margins. Bracts are oblong and persistent. Spur is absent. Leaves are paired, linear-lance shaped 15-30 cm long, 2-3 cm broad. Pseudobulbs are oblong ovoid, 5-8 cm, arising from a stout rhizome. Flowering: March-April.

Medicinal Uses:

The *juice of the pseudobulb* is applied to *boils*. This juice is also put in *wound* on the *hooves of animals*.

Tiny Dendrobium

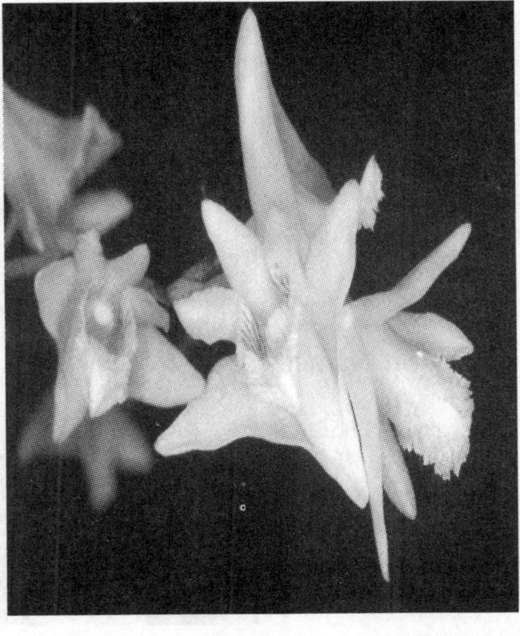

Botanical Name:
Dendrobium microbulbon

Family:
Orchidaceae **(Orchid family)**

Common Names:
Tiny Dendrobium • Marathi: *Jambhli dande amri*

Description:
Tiny Dendrobium is a small epiphytic rare orchid native to peninsular India, which can be often seen growing out of bark of trees. Pseudobulbs are small, crowded and ovoid. The plant has two leaves which are linear-oblong and pointed. Flowering stem is leafless, solitary, erect, 4-8 flowered. Bracts are nearly as long as the stalk. Flowers are white, tinged with purple. They are small, about 1-1.2 cm across, stalked. Lateral sepals are obtuse, petals narrowly arranged, nearly spoon-shaped, mentum long incurved, lip thick, side lobes broad acute, midlobe small round crenulate, disk with a channelled ridge thickened at the end.

Medicinal Uses:
Tiny Dendrobium is used in *stomachaches*, by the *tribal people of Gujarat.*

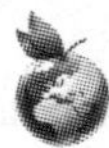

Edgeworth`s Habenaria

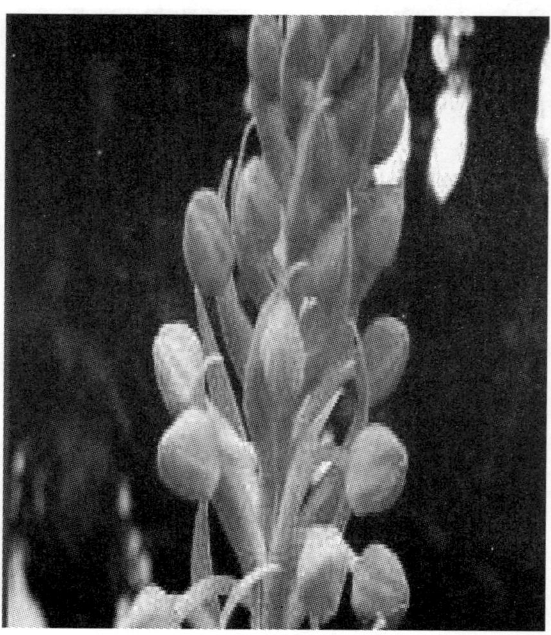

Botanical Name:
Habenaria edgeworthii

Family:
Orchidaceae **(Orchid family)**

Synonyms:
Platanthera edgeworthii

Common Names:
Edgeworth's Habenaria • Hindi: *Riddhi* • Tamil: *Riddhi* • Malayalam: *Riddhi* • Telugu: *Riddhi* • Kannada: *Riddhi* • Sanskrit: *Riddhi*

Description:
Edgeworth's Habenaria is a tuberous terrestrial orchid, growing up to 75 cm tall. It has somewhat twisted leafy stem covered with hairs. Leaves are sheathed, 2-4 in number, ovate to lance-shaped. Flowers are yellowish green deflexed in buds, in cylindrical spikes. Lip is bright yellow, entire, strap-shaped, base forming slightly channelled claw, spur longer than ovary, spreading and directed upwards usually hooked downwards towards the tip, column 2-3 mm in height. Edgeworth's Habenaria is found in the *Himalayas*, from Uttarakhand to Nepal, at altitudes of 2500-3000 m.

Medicinal Uses:
The *tubers* of Edgeworth's Habenaria are used in *Ayurvedic medicine.* The medicine goes by the name, *Riddhi.*

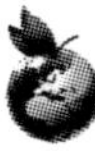

Jeevak

Botanical Name:
Malaxis acuminata

Family:
Orchidaceae **(Orchid family)**

Synonyms:
Microstylis wallichii

Common Names:
Jeevak • Hindi: *Jivak* • Tamil: *Jivakam* • Malayalam: *Jivakam* • Telugu: *Jivakamu* • Kannada: *Jivaka* • Sanskrit: *Jivakah*

Description:
Found in India, China, and South-East Asia at elevations up to to 1400 m, Jeevak is a small to medium sized, hot to warm growing terrestrial or lithophytic orchid. It occurs on highly eroded, stratified limestone cliffs and bluffs with horizontal rhizomes giving rise to rather thin, short stems, each bearing 3-5, broadly lance-like, acuminate and acute, leaves. The plant blooms in summer on an erect, 4-12 inches long, several to many flowered inflorescence with lanceolate acute floral bracts. Flowers minute, pale-yellowish green, tinged with purple, in terminal racemes. Sides of the lip produced upwards into auricles, and the apex is notched.

Medicinal Uses:
The *pseudobulbs* are *sweet*, *refrigerant*, *aphrodisiac*, *febrifuge* and *tonic*. They are useful in *haematemesis*, *fever*, *seminal weakness*, *burning sensations*, *dipsia*, *emaciation*, *tuberculosis* and *general debility*.

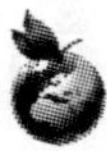

Desert Hyacinth

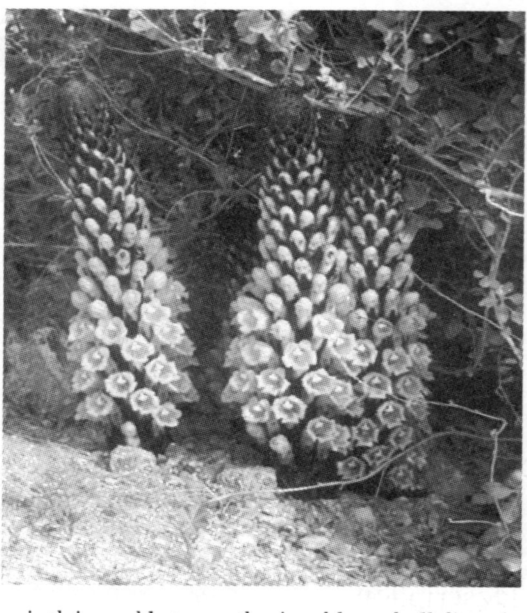

Botanical Name:
Cistanche tubulosa

Family:
Orobanchaceae **(Desert hyacinth family)**

Common Names:
Desert hyacinth, Fox radish
• Hindi: *Lonki-ka-mula*

Description:
Desert hyacinth is all-flower bearing parasite plant, growing on roots of desert shrubs. It is a rare and endangered species. Most preferred host for this parasite is *Salvadora persica.* Desert hyacinth is unable to synthesise chlorophyll directly and therefore, has *no green colouration.* It is a widely distributed annual that produces a dense pyramid spike of bright yellow flowers topped by maroon-tinted buds. Its many tiny seeds may remain dormant for years until the roots of its host plant are close enough to trigger germination. The plant is able to tolerate *saline environments* and is most found in *arid regions of Rajasthan, Punjab and Pakistan.*

Medicinal Uses:
In Taiwan, *Desert Hyacinth* is traditionally used as a *tonic drug for deficiency of the kidney* characterised by *impotence, cold sensation* in the *loins* and *knees, female sterility* and *constipation* due to *dryness of the bowel* in the senile.

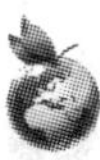

Bilimbi

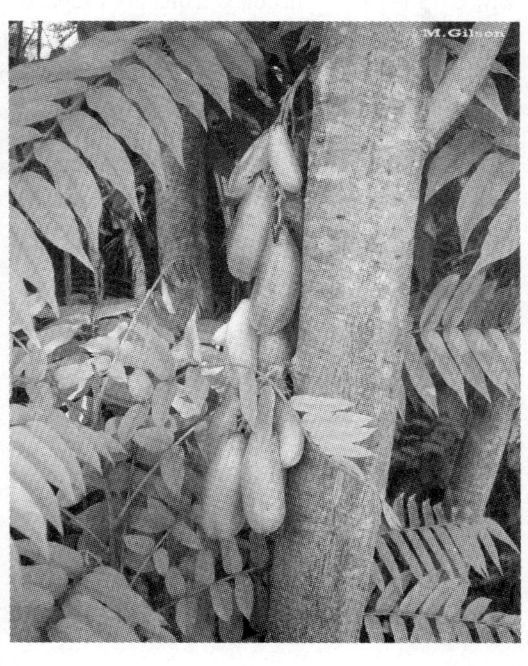

Botanical Name:
Averrhoa bilimbi

Family:
Oxalidaceae **(Wood sorrel family)**

Common Names:
Bilimbi, Cucumber-*Tree* • Hindi: *Bilimbi* • Manipuri: *Heinajom* • Marathi: *Bilambi* • Tamil: *Pulima* • Malayalam: *Vilumpi* • Telugu: *Gommareku* • Kannada: *Belambu* • Konkani: *Bimbul*

Description:
The Bilimbi tree is long-lived, reaches 5-10 m in height. Its trunk is short and quickly divides up into ramifications.

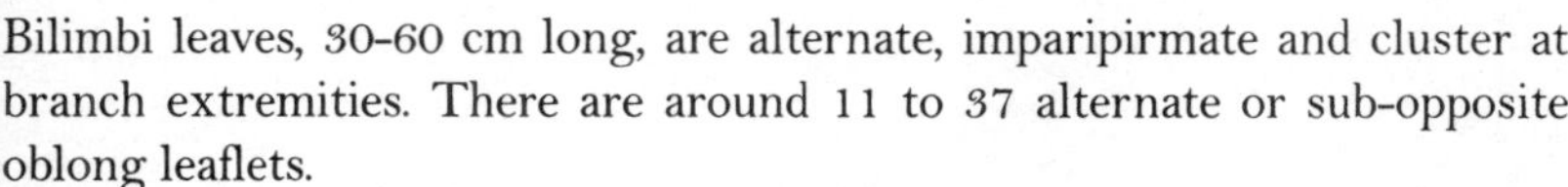

Bilimbi leaves, 30-60 cm long, are alternate, imparipirmate and cluster at branch extremities. There are around 11 to 37 alternate or sub-opposite oblong leaflets.

This Carambola relative produces very small pickle-like fruits which are borne directly on the trunk of the tree and also on the branches. The fruits are preceded by small red flowers on the trunk and branches.

Its flowers, like its fruits, are found in hairy panicles that directly emerge from the trunk as well as from the oldest, most solid branches.

The yellowish or purplish flowers are tiny, fragrant and have 5 petals. The Bilimbi fruit's form ranges from ellipsoid to almost cylindrical. Its length is 4-10 cm.

The Bilimbi is 5-sided, but in a less marked way than the Carambola. If unripe, it is bright green and crispy. It turns yellowish as it ripens. The flesh is juicy, green and extremely acidic.

The fruit's skin is glossy and very thin. The Bilimbi is too acid for eating raw but the green uncooked fruits are prepared as a relish in Suriname.

Originated seemingly from the Moluccas, in India, where it is usually found in gardens, the Bilimbi has gone wild in the warmest regions of the country.

Medicinal Uses:

In Malaysia, the *leaves of Bilimbi* are used as a treatment for *venereal diseases.* A *leaf decoction* is taken as a medicine to relieve *rectal inflammation.* It seems to be effective against *coughs and thrush too.*

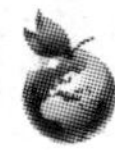

Opium Poppy

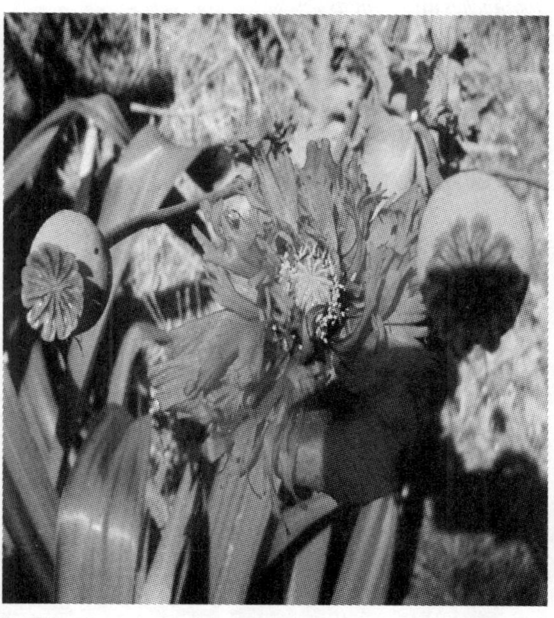

Botanical Name:

Papaver somniferum

Family:

Papaveraceae **(Poppy family)**

Common Names:

Opium Poppy • Hindi: *Afim*

Description:

Poppy is an annual herb native to Southeastern Europe and western Asia. Also known as opium poppy, the species is cultivated extensively in many countries, including Iran, Turkey, Holland, Poland, Romania, Czechoslovakia, Yugoslavia, India, Canada, and many Asian, Central and South American countries.

Reaching a height of 1.2 metres, the erect plant can have white, pink, red, or purple flowers. Seeds range in colour from white to a slate shade that is called blue in commercial classifications.

A latex containing several important alkaloids is obtained from immature seed capsules one to three weeks after flowering. Incisions are made in the walls of the green seed pods, and the milky exudation is collected and dried.

Opium and the isoquinoline alkaloids, morphine, codeine, noscapine, papaverine and thebaine are isolated from the dried materials.

The poppy seeds and fixed oil that can be expressed from the seeds are not narcotic, because they develop after the capsule has lost the opium-yielding potential.

Medicinal Uses:

Poppy is one of the most important medicinal plants. Traditionally, the dry opium was considered an *astringent, antispasmodic, aphrodisiac, diaphoretic, expectorant, hypnotic, narcotic,* and sedative. Poppy has been used against *toothaches* and *coughs.*

The ability of opium from poppy to serve as an *analgesic* is well known. Opium and derivatives of opium are used in the *pharmaceutical industry* as narcotic analgesics, hypnotics and sedatives.

Opium and the drugs derived from opium are addictive and can have toxicological effects.

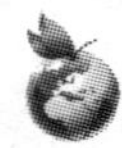

Love in a Mist

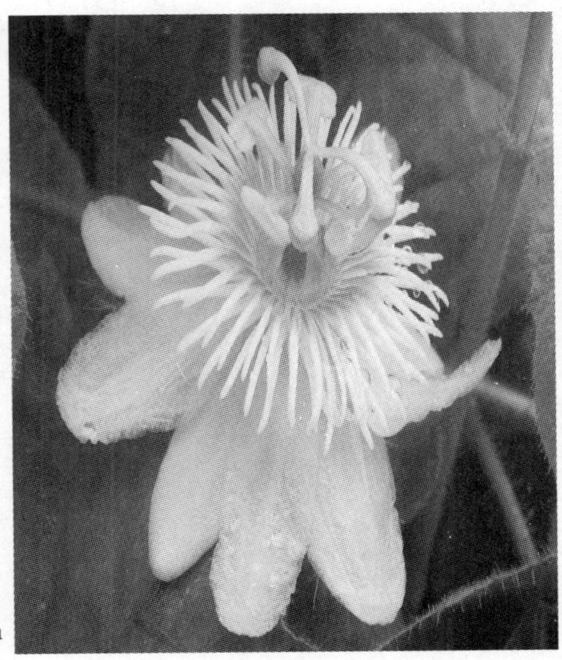

Botanical Name:

Passiflora foetida

Family:

Passifloraceae **(Passion flower family)**

Common Names:

Love-in-a-mist, Stinking passionflower • Hindi: *Jhumka lata* • Bengali: *Jhumka lota* • Marathi: Vel-ghani • Kannada: *Kukkiballi* • Malayalam: *Poochapalam* • Telugu: *Tellajumiki*

Description:

Love-in-a-mist is a *creeping vine* which has an edible fruits and leaves that have a *mildly rank aroma.* It is native to northern South America and the West Indies. The stems are thin, wiry and woody, covered with sticky yellow hairs.

The leaves are three-to five-lobed and viscid-hairy. They give off an unpleasant odour when crushed. The flowers are white to pale cream coloured, about 5-6 cm diameter.

The fruit is globose, 2-3 cm diameter, yellowish-orange to red when ripe, and has numerous black seeds embedded in the pulp; the fruit are eaten and the seeds dispersed by birds.

The bracts of this plant serve as *insect traps,* but it is as yet unknown whether the plant digests and gains nourishment from the trapped insects or if it merely uses the bracts as a defensive mechanism to protect its flowers and fruits. This is still an issue of debate and research among carnivorous plant enthusiasts.

Medicinal Uses:

This species can be helpful in *treating digestive problems,* including *dyspepsia* and *diarrhoea*; or used as an *astringent and expectorant* for nervous conditions and spasms.

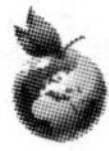

Bara Gokhru

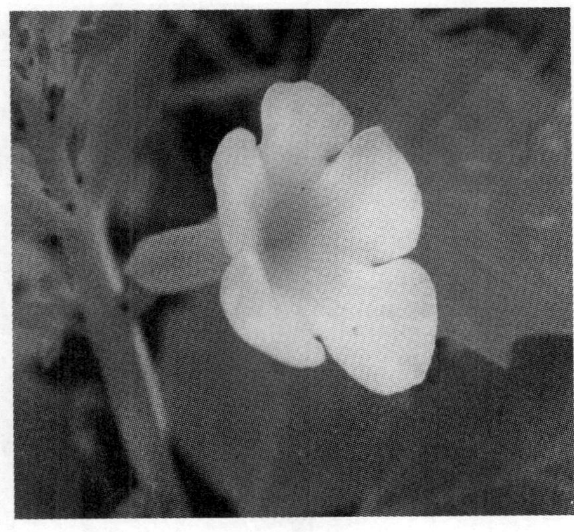

Botanical Name:
Pedalium murex

Family:
Pedaliaceae **(Sesame family)**

Common Names:
Large Caltrops • Hindi: *Bara Gokhru* • Kannada: *Ane neggilu* • Malayalam: *Ananerinnil* • Tamil: *Yanai nerunjil* • Oriya: *Gokhara* • Marathi: *Gokhura* • Gujarati: *Kadva gokhru*

Description:
A shrubby stiff stemmed herb, native to India, grown for reputed medicinal and other uses. It is diffused annually, much branched, spreading, succulent, glandular, up to 60 cm tall. Roots similar to turmeric in colour. Leaves simple, opposite, ovate or oblong-obovate, 1-4.5 cm long, irregularly and coarsely crenate-serrate. Yellow flowers 1.5-2 cm across, stalk 1-2 mm long, increasing up to 4 mm in fruits. Sepals 2 mm long; teeth linear, scaly outside and persistent. Petals fused into a broad tube, 1-3 cm long; lobes obtuse. Stamens 0.5-1 cm long; anthers kidney shaped. The four angled seed is with five extremely sharp spines. *It is an important famine food - leaves eaten as vegetables.*

Medicinal Uses:
Leaves are *antibilious. Seeds* are *demulcant, diuretic, tonic, muscilaginous* and *aphrodesiac.* Used in *male impotence, gonorrhoea* and *incontinence.*

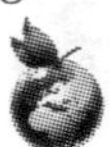

Mousetail Plant

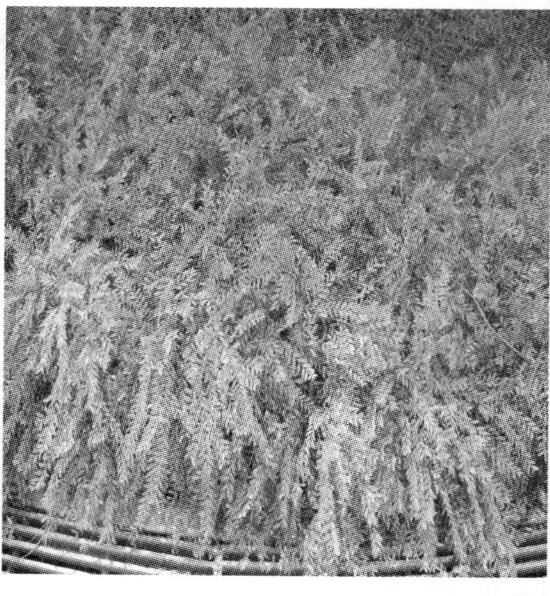

Botanical Name:
Phyllanthus myrtifolius

Family:
Phyllanthaceae **(Amla family)**

Common Names:
Mousetail Plant, Myrtle-leaved Leaf Flower

Description:
Mousetail Plant is a *small shrub* about 50 cm tall with tiny inverted-lance shaped leaves and small, slender, pendulous red flowers which probably inspired the name, Mousetail Plant. Branches are cylindrical, branchlets wing-angled, angles rough. Alternately arranged leaves are inverted-lance shaped, 1.2-1.6 cm long and 3.5-4.5 mm wide, leathery, smooth, tip not sharp pointed. Flowers are borne in several-flowered fascicles in leaf axils. Flowers are typically longer than the leaves and hang down by slender, red filament-like stalks, ending in a roundish bowl-like flower. Fruits are capsules, 2 mm long and 3 mm wide. Mousetail Plant is native to Sri Lanka. It is grown as an ornament, particularly as a *bonsai* in North - East India. Flowering: May-August.

Medicinal Uses:
Mousetail Plant is grown as a *medicinal plant in China.*

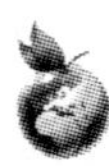

Black-Honey Shrub

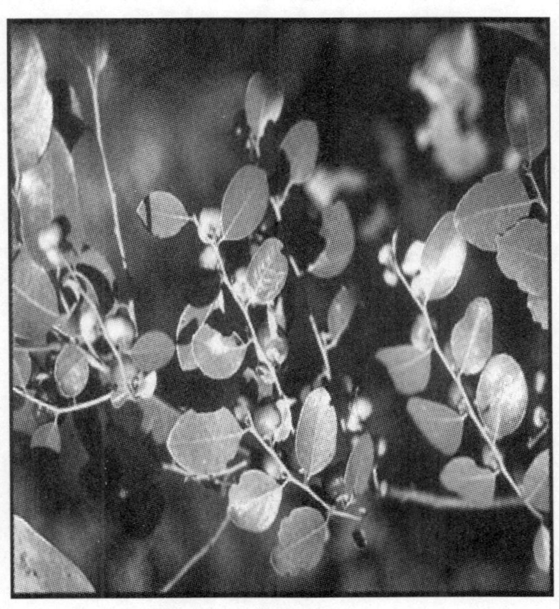

Botanical Name:
Phyllanthus reticulatus

Family:
Phyllanthaceae **(Amla family)**

Synonyms:
Kirganelia reticulata, Anisonema reticulatum, Cicca reticulata, Diasperus reticulates

Common Names:
Black-Honey Shrub, Black-berried featherfoil, Potato-bush, Netted-leaved leaf-flower • Assamese: *Amlakhi* • Bengali: *Panjuli* • Gujarati: *Kamboi* • Hindi: *Kale madhu ka per, Makhi, Panjuli* • Kannada: *Karihuli* • Konkani: *Panpoi* • Malayalam: *Mirnelli* • Marathi: *Panjuli, Panpoi, Pavari* • Oriya: *Bala datun, Bonoti-hudi, Jandaki, Jojangi, Phajoli* • Sanskrit: *Krishna-kamboji* • Tamil: *Civappu-p-pula, Karu-nelli, Kattu-k-kila-nelli, Pula* • Telugu: *Nallapuli*

Description:
Black-Honey Shrub is usually a much-branched somewhat climbing shrub, rarely a small tree.

Leaves are ovate-oblong to elliptic, 1-5 cm long, 0.7-3 cm wide, produced on short lateral branchlets, looking like leaflets of a compound leaf.

Flowers are borne in clusters on short axillary branchlets, small, yellowish, sexes separate on the same plant, flowering before or with the new leaves.

The flowering shoots and pedicels are covered in short, velvety hairs. Fruits are berry-like, 4–6 mm across, blackish when ripe. Flowering: March-July.

Medicinal Uses:

The *leaves and roots* are used as a medicine for fractures and traumatic injuries.

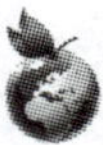

Chamber Bitter

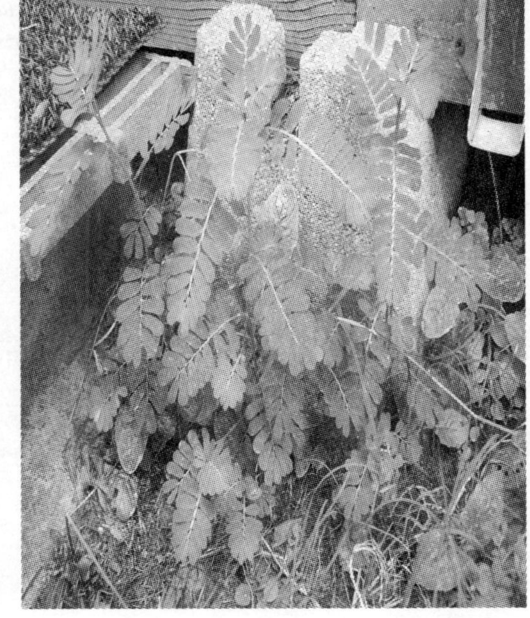

Botanical Name:
Phyllanthus urinaria

Family:
Phyllanthaceae **(Amla family)**

Synonyms:
Phyllanthus leprocarpus

Common Names:
Chamber Bitter, Common leaf-flower, Shatterstone, Stone-breaker Herb • Hindi: *Hajarmani, Lal bhuinanwalah* • Manipuri: *Chakpa-heikru* • Marathi: *Laal bhooyiavali* • Tamil: *Civappu kilanelli, Cirukilanelli* • Malayalam: *Chirukizhukanelli, Chukannakizhanelli* • Telugu: *Erra usirika* • Kannada: *Kempu kirunelli, Kempu nelanelli* • Bengali: *Hazarmani* • Sanskrit: *Bhumyamalaki, Ujjhata* • Nepali: *Kanthad*

Description:
Chamber Bitter is a small annual herb growing up to 2 ft tall. Leaves are alternately arranged along the erect, red stem, resembling those of the mimosa tree, disposed in two ranges.

However, the leaves are not compound, but simple. The leaves are oblong or oblong-obovate, 7-18 mm long, 3-7 mm wide, rounded with a sharp point., obliquely rounded at base, nearly stalkless and pale beneath.

The leaves are large at the tip and smaller towards the petioles. When touched, the leaves fold in automatically. Flowers are greenish white, minute and appear at axiles of the leaves, as well as the seed capsules.

Numerous small green-red fruits, round and smooth, are found along the underside of the stems.

Medicinal Uses:

It is used against *colic,* and as an effective remedy to eliminate *gall bladder* and *kidney stones, urinary tract infections,* bladder inflammations and for other *kidney and liver problems* in general, such as *acute and chronic Hepatitis B,* which explains the origin of its species name, *urinaria.*

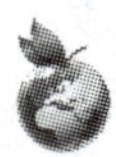

Guinea Henweed

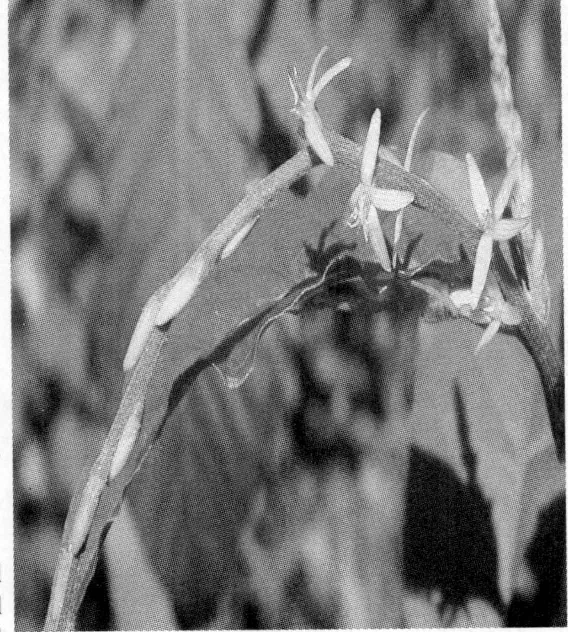

Botanical Name:

Petiveria alliacea

Family:

Phytolaccaceae
(Pokeweed family)

Synonyms:

Mapa graveolens, Petiveria corrientina, Petiveria foetida, Petiveria graveolens

Common Names:

Guinea Henweed, Anamu, Garlic weed

Description:

Guinea Henweed is a deeply rooted herbacious perennial shrub native to tropical areas of Africa, South and Central America and the Caribbean islands.

It has now naturalised in India, and it grows up to 1 m tall, having velvety to smooth stems.

The roots and leaves have a strong, garlic-like odour which taints the milk and meat of animals that graze on it.

It produces dark green leathery leaves that lie close to the ground and tall spikes lined with small white flowers that sway above the leaves.

Leaves are elliptic to oblong or obovate, to 20 × 7 cm, with 0.4–2 cm long stalks. Base is acute to wedge-shaped, tip is narrow or acute to obtuse or rounded in shape.

Flowers are regularly spaced, with white or greenish to pinkish, linear-lance shaped to linear-oblong sepals, about 3.5-6 mm long.

Medicinal Uses:

Guinea Henweed has been widely used to treat an *astounding range of medical conditions both in humans and in animals* including: *venereal diseases*, an *antiseptic, arthritis, pain, cancers, womb inflammations, diuretic, decoagulant, cold, snake-bites,* flu, cods, hysteria, paralysis, fever, rabies, etc., to treat arrow poison in Brazil and as a *bat and insect repellent.*

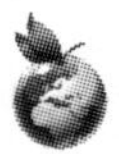

Chir Pine

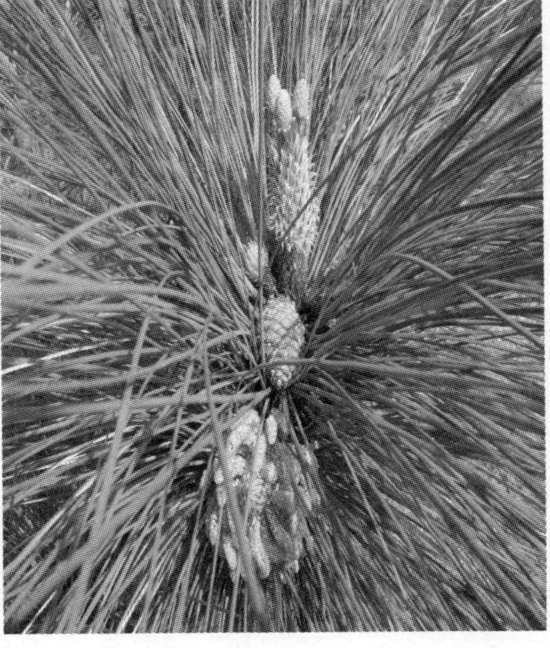

Botanical Name:

Pinus roxburghii

Family:

Pinaceae **(Pine family)**

Synonyms:

Pinus longifolia

Common Names:

Chir pine, Himalayan longleaf pine • Hindi: *Chir* • Manipuri: *Wuchan*

Description:

Among the principal pines found in India, Chir pine is the most important. Native to the Himalayas, it is good as a *street tree* too. This is one of the least exacting of the *Himalayan trees* growing sometimes on bare rocks, where only a few species are capable of existing.

It is a *resinous tree* capable of yielding resin continuously provided the r*ill method of tapping* is adopted. Erect, round-headed evergreen tree with one or more trunks. Grows at moderate rate to 30 ft., with spread of 20 ft at maturity.

The bark is red-brown, thick and deeply fissured at the base of the trunk, thinner and flaky in the upper crown.

The leaves are needle-like, in fascicles of three, very slender, 20-35 cm long, and distinctly yellowish green. The flowers are monoecious (individual flowers are either male or female, but both sexes can be found on the same plant) and are pollinated by wind.

The cones are ovoid conic, 12-24 cm long and 5-8 cm broad at the base when closed, green at first and ripening glossy chestnut-brown when 24 months old. They open slowly over the next year or so.

Medicinal Uses:

The turpentine obtained from the *resin* of all *pine trees* is *antiseptic, diuretic, rubefacient* and *vermifuge.*

It is a valuable remedy used internally in the treatment of *kidney and bladder complaints* and is used both internally and as a rub and steam bath in the treatment of *rheumatic affections.*

It is also very *beneficial to the respiratory system* and so is useful *in treating diseases of the mucous membranes* and *respiratory complaints,* such as *coughs, colds, influenza* and Tuberculosis. Externally, it is a very beneficial treatment for a variety of *skin complaints, wounds, sores, burns, boils,* etc and is used in the form of liniment plasters, poultices, herbal steam baths and inhalers.

The wood is diaphoretic and stimulant. It is useful in treating burning of the body, cough, fainting and ulcers.

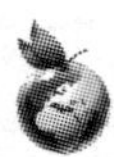

Shiny Bush

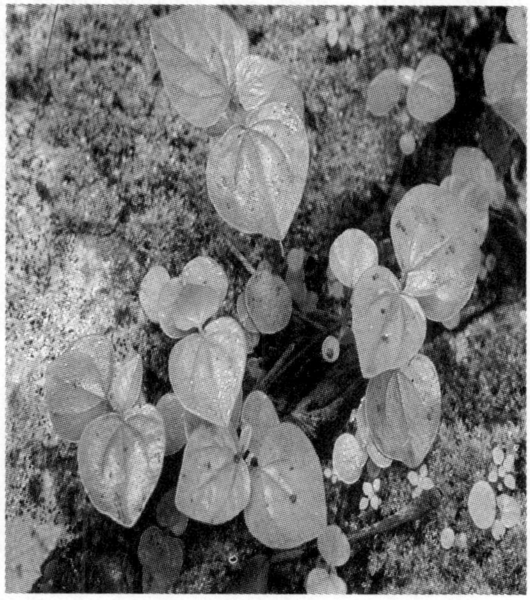

Botanical Name:
Peperomia pellucida

Family:
Piperaceae **(Pepper family)**

Synonyms:
Peperomia exigua, Peperomia translucens, Piper pellicudum

Common Names:
Shiny Bush, Slate pencil plant, Pepper elder, Rat's ear, Shiny bush, silverbush • Malayalam: *Mashitandu chedi* • Assamese: *Pononoa* • Sanskrit: *Toyakandha, Varshabhoo*

Description:
Shiny bush is *a common fleshy annual herb,* growing by roadside and in wasteland. Stems are translucent pale green, erect or ascending, usually 15-45 cm long, internodes usually 3-8 cm long, hairless.

Fleshy leaves are heart shaped, shiny light green, 1.5-4 cm long, 1-3.3 cm wide. It has very small bi-sexual flowers growing in the form of cord-like spikes, 3-6 cm long, arising from the leaf axils.

The fruits are also very small, round to oblong, ridged, first green later black. They have one single seed. Shiny bush has a mustard like odour.

The plant can be utilised as a vegetable and in salads. Shiny Bush is native to South America, but widely naturalised and cultivated.

Medicinal Uses:

In South America, the Shiny Bush is used medicinally. A solution of the *fresh juice of stem and leaves* is used against *eye inflammation.*

It has also been applied against *coughing, fever, common cold, headache, sore throat, diarrhoea, against kidney*-and *prostate problems* and against *high blood pressure.* Shiny bush is also used in *Ayurvedic medicine.*

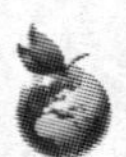

Long Pepper

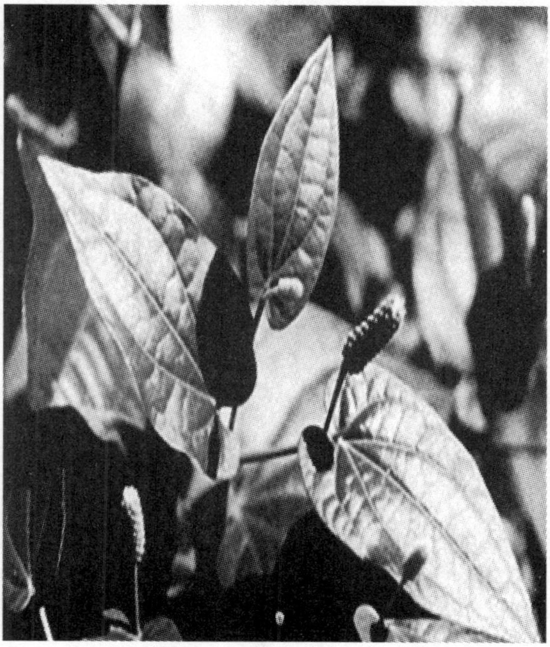

Botanical Name:
Piper longum

Family:
Piperaceae **(Pepper family)**

Common Names:
Long Pepper, Indian long pepper • Hindi: *Pipli* • Marathi: *Pimpli* • Tamil: *Tippili* • Malayalam: *Tippali* • Telugu: *Pippallu* • Kannada: *Kandan Lippili* • Konkani: *Pipli* • Urdu: *Pipul* • Gujarati: *Pipari* • Sanskrit: *Pippali, Magadhi*

Description:
Long Pepper is a climber, of South Asian origin (Deccan peninsula), cultivated for its fruits, which is usually dried and used as a *spice* for seasoning.

Long pepper is a close relative of the black pepper plant, and has a similar, though generally hotter, taste. The word, pepper itself is derived from the Sanskrit word for long pepper, *pippali.*

It is a slender, aromatic, climber with perennial woody roots, creeping and jointed stems, and fleshy fruits embedded in the spikes.

Leaves are numerous, 6.3 to 9.0 cm, broadly ovate or oblong-oval, dark green and shining above, pale and dull beneath.

The older leaves are dentate, dark in colour and heart shaped. The younger leaf is ovate in shape and contains 5 veins on them.

Flowers are monoceous and male and female flowers are borne on different plants. Male flower stalk is about 1 to 3 inch long and female flower stalk is ½ to 1 inch long.

Fruit is long. When it ripes it attains red colour and when it dries it attains black colour. It is one inch in diameter. The plant flowers in rains and fruits in early winters.

Medicinal Uses:

Pippali is certainly one of the most widely used of all *Ayurvedic herbs.* It is one of the best herbs for enhancing *digestion, assimilation* and *metabolism of the foods* we eat.

It is also highly prized for its ability to enhance assimilation and potency of herbs in a synergistic formula (this is called the *Yogavahi effect*).

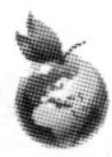

Lal Chitrak

Botanical Name:
Plumbago indica

Family:
Plumbaginaceae
(Plumbago family)

Common Names:
Plumbago, Scarlet leadwort • Hindi: *Lal chitrak* • Oriya: *Ogni* • Bengali: *Rakt-chitrak* • Tamil: *Akkini* • Gujarati: *Kalochitrak* • Kannada: *Chitramulika* • Malayalam: *Kotuveli* • Konkani: *Tambdi chitrak*

Description:
Lal Chitrak is a plant commonly cultivated in gardens throughout India. This winter flowering plant begins to show off its soft red, festive colours in time for winters. A nice change from the traditional poinsettia, this Indian native continues to flower for months to come.

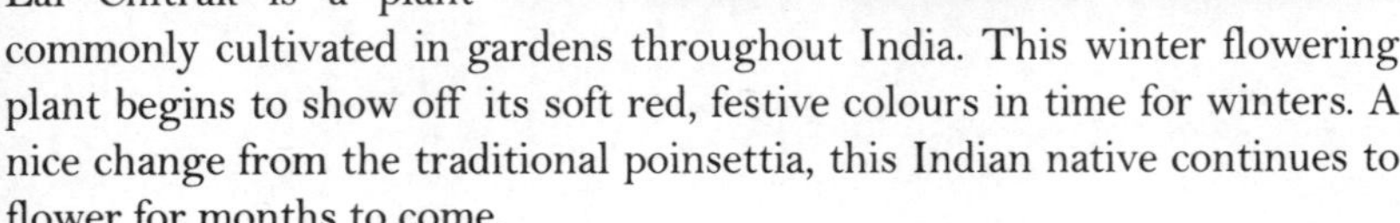

Lal Chitrak makes an outstanding container plant for a sunny window. Watch with fascination how the flowers keep emerging on the same flower spike from winter until spring.

This is an erect or spreading, more or less branched, herbaceous or half-woody plant 1.5 meters or less in height. The leaves are ovate to oblong-ovate, 8 to 13 centimeters long, slightly drooping, and smooth, with entire, undulate or wavy margins, pointed or blunt tip, and pointed base.

The spikes are 15 to 30 centimeters long. The calyx is tubular, 8 to 10 millimeters long, and covered with stalked, sticky glands.

The corolla is bright red, the tube is slender and about 2.5 centimeters long, and the limb, which spreads, is about 3 cm in diameter.

Medicinal Uses:

The *root* is *acrid*, *vesicant*, *abortifacient* and a *stimulant*. Applied in *bland oil*, it is used *externally or internally* in *rheumatism* and *paralytic afflictions.*

The *root* is a powerful *sialogogue* and a *remedy for secondary syphilis*, *leprosy* and *leucoderma*. The *milky juice of the plant* is used in *ophthalmia* and in *scabies.*

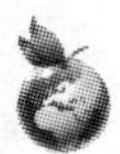

Chitrak

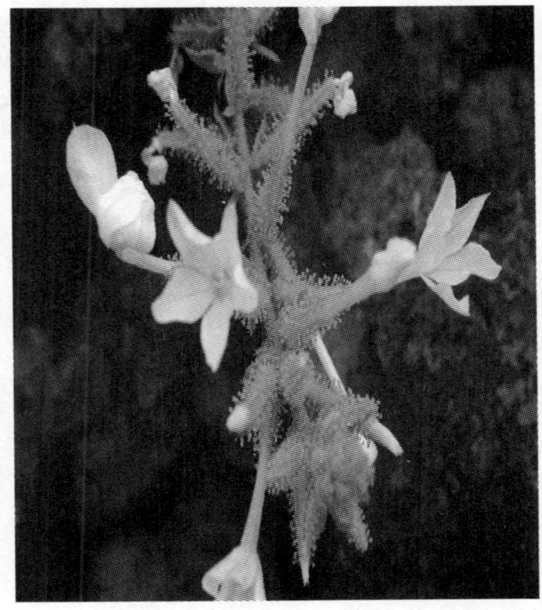

Botanical Name:
Plumbago zeylanica

Family:
Plumbaginaceae
(Plumbago family)

Common Names:
Chitrak, Plumbago, White leadwort • Hindi: *Chitrak* • Manipuri: *Telhidak angouba* • Tamil: *Chittiramoolam Karimai* • Malayalam: *Vellakoduveli* • Kannada: *Chitramulika* • Bengali: *Safaid-sitarak* • Oriya: *Ogni*

Description:
Chitrak is a herb that grows wild in India and has been used by rural and tribal people for hundreds of years as a traditional system of medicine. Chitrak is native to South-east Asia. It is a much branched, evergreen shrub that reaches about 6 feet in nature.

Dark green leaves are ovate to 6 inches long by half as wide. They are fast growing plants, but their size is easily controlled by pot size and pruning.

The flowers are white in showy dense racemes and will flower all year long. Individual flowers are up to ½ inch (a bit more than 1 cm) across. Chitrak needs full sun to partial shade with intermediate to warm temperatures.

After flowering, the plants should be cut back to keep them growing vigorously. The fruits are like a small cocklebur with glue on the soft spines and they will stick to anything.

The root and root bark and seeds are used medicinally as a stimulant, caustic, digestion, antiseptic, anti-parasitic.

Chitrak is propagated by *cuttings, division of older plants* or by *seeds.*

Medicinal Uses:

Chitrak is used in treating *intestinal troubles, dysentery, leucoderma, inflammation, piles, bronchitis, itching, diseases* of the *liver*, and *consumption.*

The leaves of this herb work well for treating *laryngitis, rheumatism, diseases of the spleen, ring worm, scabies,* and it acts as an *aphrodisiac.*

A *tincture of the root bark* is used as an *anti-periodic.* The Chitrak root helps *improve digestion* and it *stimulates the appetite.* The Chitrak root is also an *acro-narcotic poison* that can cause *an abortion.*

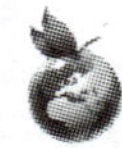

Crowfoot Grass

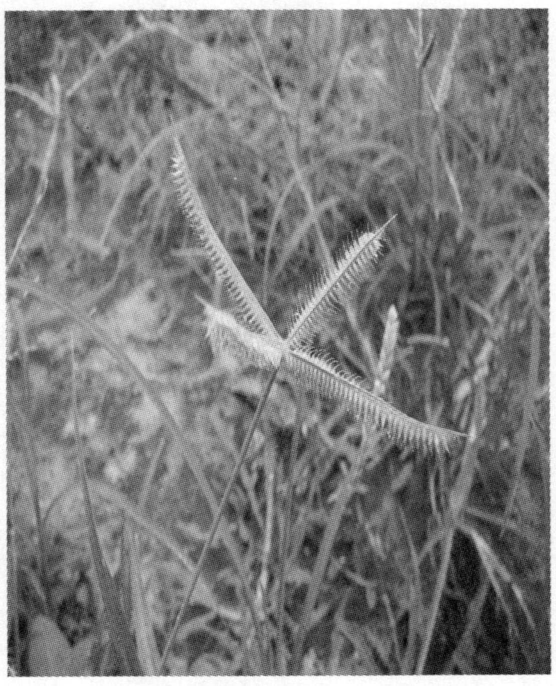

Botanical Name:
Dactyloctenium aegyptium

Family:
Poaceae **(Grass family)**

Synonyms:
Eleusine aegyptiaca

Common Names:
Crowfoot Grass, Beach wiregrass, Coast button grass, Comb fringe grass, Duck grass, Durban crowfoot, Egyptian fingergrass, Egyptian grass, Finger comb grass, Four-finger grass • Hindi: *Makra* • Manipuri: *Pungphai*

Description:
Crowfoot Grass is a slender to moderately robust, spreading annual herb, with wiry stems, that bend and root at the lower nodes, with tips that may rise to about 2 ft in height.

It is a very common weed of open spaces and wasteland. Leaves are typically grass-like, 2-30 cm long, 2-9 mm wide, with blades and sheaths that are without hair.

Leaf margins have long, stiff hairs. Flowers arise in 1-7 spikes, 1-6.2 cm long, 3-7 mm wide, at the tip of stems. Seed head resembles a crow's foot, hence the Common Names.

Crowfoot Grass is native to Africa, but naturalised world-wide.

Medicinal Uses:

In Manipur, the juice of fresh plants is prescribed in *fevers. Decoction* of the plant is given in *small pox.*

Perennial Buckwheat

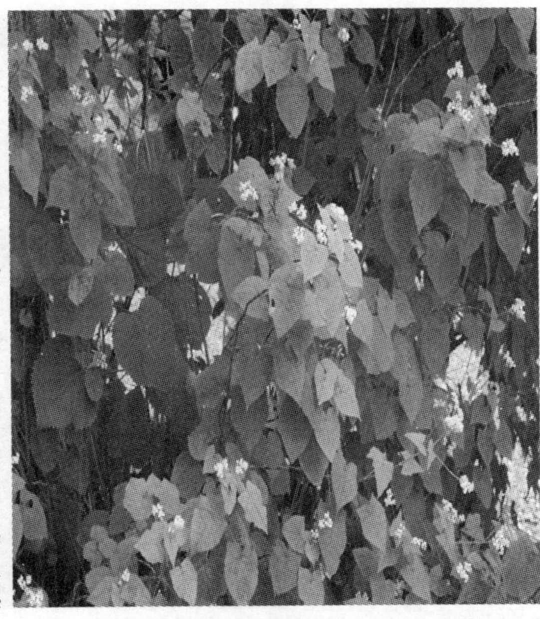

Botanical Name:
Fagopyrum dibotrys

Family:
Polygonaceae **(Knotweed family)**

Common Names:
Perennial Buckwheat, Tall Buckwheat

Description:
Perennial growing to 1m by 2m at a fast rate. It is frost tender. It is in flower in September. The flowers are monoecious (individual flowers are either male or female, but both sexes can be found on the same plant) and are pollinated by Bees and flies. We rate it 4 out of 5 for usefulness. The plant prefers light (sandy), medium (loamy) and heavy (clay) soils, requires well-drained soil and can grow in heavy clay and nutritionally poor soils. The plant prefers acid, neutral and basic (alkaline) soils. It can grow in semi-shade (light woodland) or no shade. It requires dry or moist soil.

Medicinal Uses:
The whole plant is *anodyne, anthelmintic, antiphlogistic, carminative, depurative* and *febrifuge.* It stimulates *blood circulation.* A *decoction* is used in the treatment of traumatic injuries, lumbago, menstrual irregularities, in *purulent infections, snake and insect bites.*

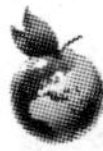

Oriental Pepper

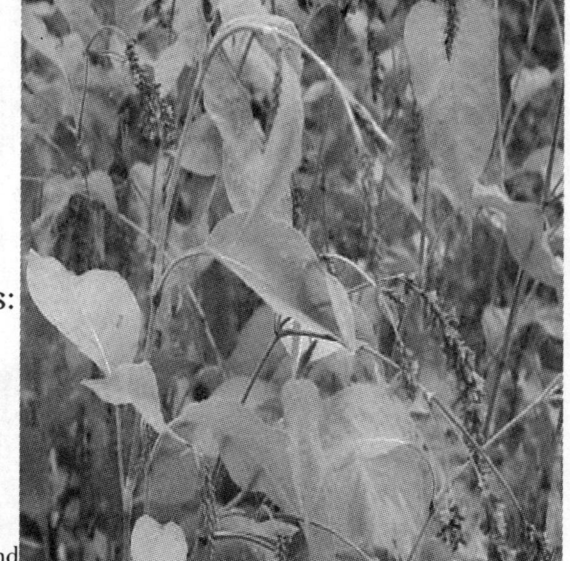

Botanical Name:
Polygonum orientale

Family:
Polygonaceae
(Knotweed family)

Synonyms:
Persicaria orientalis

Common Names:
Oriental Pepper, Prince's feather, Tall Persicaria • Hindi: Machoti • Bengali: Bishkatala

Description:
Oriental Pepper is found in open, wet places along streams at low and medium altitudes. It also occurs in China to Japan and southward to Australia. The plant is a branching annual, 30-100 cm in height. The leaves are long-stalked, ovate or ovate-cordate, 15-20 cm long, 5-12 cm wide, and covered with soft, silky, grey hairs. The racemes are cylindric, laxly panicled, and 8-13 cm long. The flowers are white. The nut is about 3 mm in diameter, rounded, black, and shining. There is variety of this plant with rose-pink flowers, which is widely cultivated in the West as a garden plant, and is called *Kiss Me Over The Garden Gate.*

Medicinal Uses:
The nuts are prescribed in tuberculosis, swellings and in flatulence.

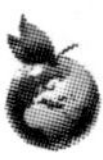

Arrowleaf Dock

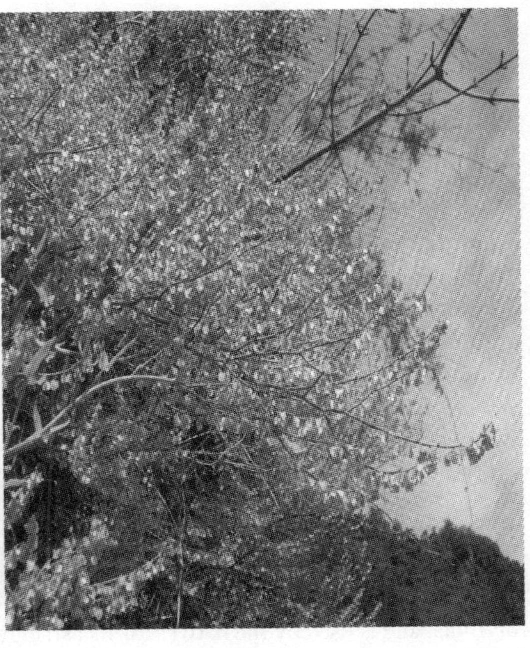

Botanical Name:

Rumex hastatus

Family:

Polygonaceae **(Knotweed family)**

Common Names:

Arrowleaf Dock, Yellow Sock, Curled Sock • Hindi: *Churki, churka*• Urdu: *Khatti Buti*

Description:

Arrowleaf Dock is a fairly common small shrub, growing on dry slopes, rocks and walls between 700-2500 m, typically in north-Indian hill stations. It is a bushy shrub with many ascending stems. Stems woody at base, leaves narrow and arrow shaped with a pair of narrow spreading basal lobe. Leaves vary a lot in length and breadth. The stems have numerous thin branches with terminal very slender clusters of distant whorls of tiny greenish pink or pinkish green flowers. Flowers very small, flower stalk lengthening in fruit. Leaves broadly triangular, stalked, fruit pinkish. Flowering: June-October.

Medicinal Uses:

The *leaf extract* of the plant is applied on *wounds and cuts* to *check bleeding*. The Plant is also believed to relieve from *suffering of nettle sting*. The root is *laxative alternative, tonic,* and *anti-rheumatic* and can be used in skin disease.

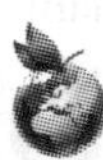

Nepal Dock

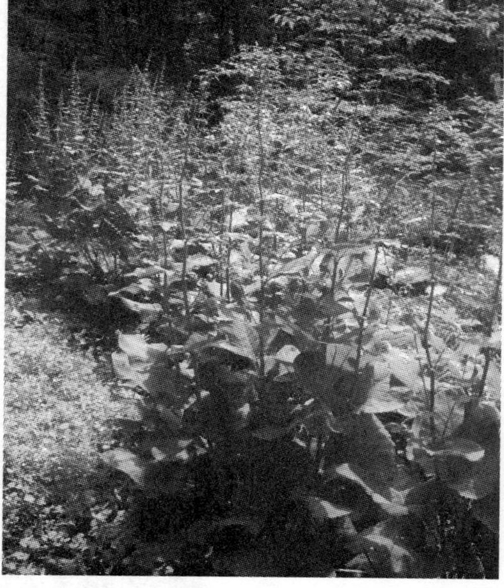

Botanical Name:

Rumex nepalensis

Family:

Polygonaceae **(Knotweed family)**

Common Names:

Nepal Dock • Assamese: *Pahari palang* • Bengali: *Pahari palang* • Hindi: *Amlya, Amlora, Bhilmora, Malori, Jangli palak* • Manipuri: *Torongkhongchak* • Tamil: *Sukkankeerai*

Description:

This plant grows abundantly in many parts of India, and is used by the natives for its astringent qualities, and for dyeing purposes. These are erect plants with long tap roots. The fleshy to leathery leaves form a basal rosette at the root. The basal leaves may be different from those near the inflorescence. The inconspicuous flowers are carried above the leaves in whorl-like clusters. The fertile flowers are mostly hermaphrodite, or they can be functionally male or female. The flowers and seeds grow on long clusters at the top of a stalk emerging from the basal rosette. Each seed is an 3-sided achene. Plants can contain quite high levels of oxalic acid, which is what gives the leaves of many members of this genus an acid-lemon flavour.

Medicinal Uses:

The leaf extract is applied to *skin sores. Leaf infusion* is given in *colic and* applied to *syphilitic ulcers. Leaves* are rubbed on the *affected part for relief from irritation* caused by the Bichchhoo plant.

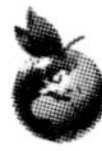

Arrow Leaf Pondweed

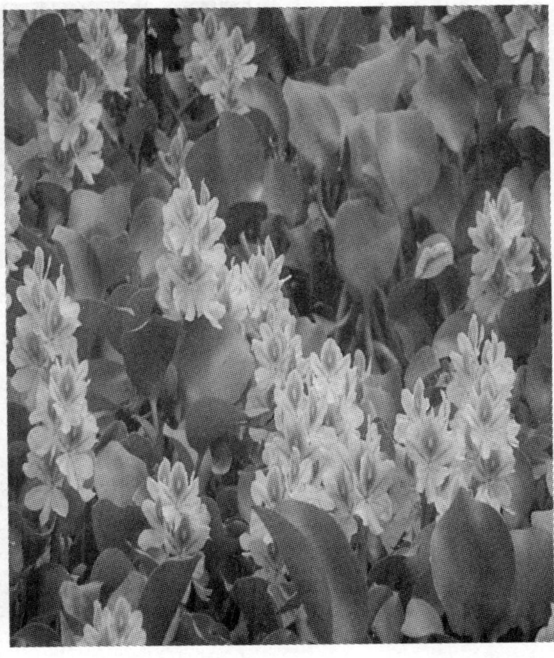

Botanical Name:
Monochoria hastata

Family:
Pontederiaceae
(Pickerel weed family)

Common Names:
Arrow Leaf Pondweed, Arrow-leaf monochoria, Hastate-leaf pondweed, Monochoria • Hindi: *Launkia* • Bengali: *Nukha*

Description:
Arrow-leaf Pondweed is an emergent aquatic herb with stems approximately 0.7-1.2 m long. The basal leaves are arrow-shaped. The inflorescence of 25- 60 flowers is in a dense spike 6-9 cm long. The flowers are 13-16 mm long, purple or whitish. One anther is coloured blue, c. 6 mm long, the other 5 anthers are yellow and c. 4 mm long. The seed capsule is 7 mm long, and 5-6 mm diameter. This species occurs in India, Sri Lanka and SE Asia, extending to New Guinea and Australia. Arrow-leaf Pondweed is often grown as an ornamental in water gardens, and the entire plant except its roots is eaten in India. Flowering: March–June.

Medicinal Uses:
The plant is considered an *alterative, tonic* and *cooling agent.* The juice of the leaves is applied to *boils.* The *rhizomes* are *powdered with charcoal* and used for *scurf.*

Oval Leaf Pondweed

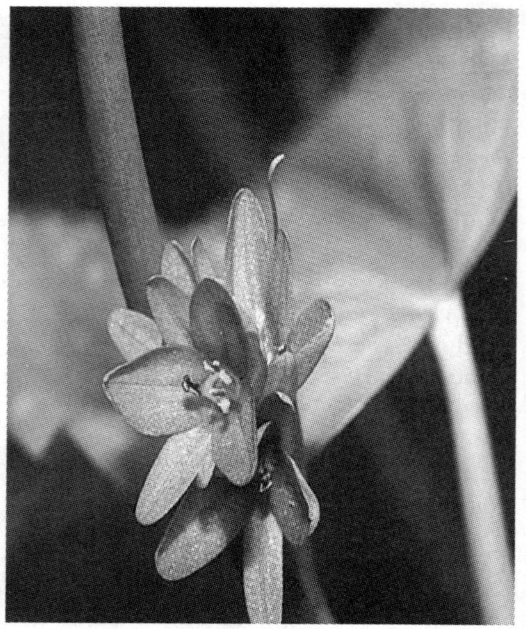

Botanical Name:

Monochoria vaginalis

Family:

Pontederiaceae **(Pickerel weed family)**

Common Names:

Oval Leaf Pondweed, Oval Leaf Monochoria, Marshy betelvine • Hindi: *Nanka, Indivar* • Marathi: *Nelat-phal* • Tamil: *Karimkuvalam* • Malayalam: *Karinkuvvalam* • Telugu: *Nirakancha* • Kannada: *Neelothpala* • Bengali: *Nukha* • Assamese: *Nara meteka* • Sanskrit: *Indivarah*

Description:

Oval Leaf Pondweed is an attached aquatic annual or perennial herb with emersed leaves, to 50 cm tall. More widespread than *M. hastata*, it is a serious weed of rice fields.

Leaves variable - 2-12.5 cm long, 0.5-10 cm wide, in very young plants without lamina; leaves of somewhat older plants with a floating linear or lanceolate blade; leaves of still older plants, ovate-oblong to broadly ovate, sharply acuminate, the base heart-shaped or rounded, shiny, deep green in colour.

Inflorescence spikelike, basally opposite the sheath of the floral leaf, with a large bract arising from a thickened bundle on leaf stalk, about two-thirds of the way up the stalk from the base.

Flowers 3-25, opening simultaneously or in quick succession, on pedicels 4-25 mm long. Petals six, violet or lilac blue, spreading at flowering, afterwards spirally contorted.

As is typical of many aquatic annuals, plant size, leaf shape and flower number are highly variable in relation to the amount of water.

The entire plant (except the roots) is eaten as a vegetable in India, and the roots are used medicinally. Flowering: August-March.

Medicinal Uses:

The oval Leaf Pondweed is used in *Ayurvedic, Unani* and *Folklore* medicines. The *root* is used for *toothaches* and the bark is eaten with sugar for *asthma.*

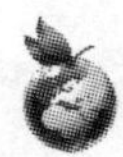

Common Rock Jasmine

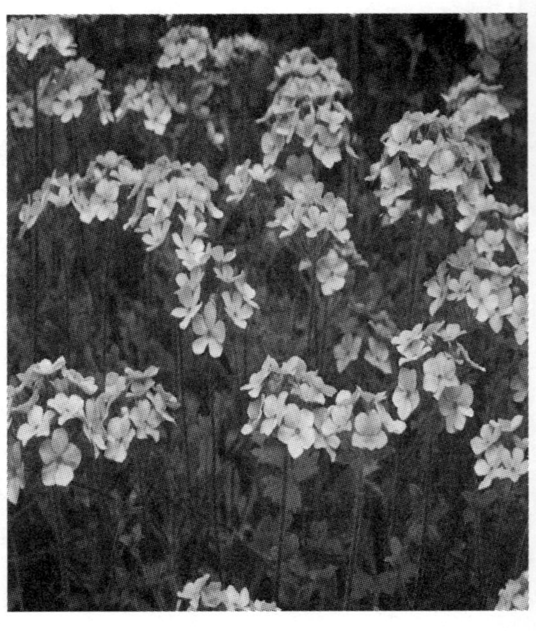

Botanical Name:
Androsace sarmentosa

Family:
Primulaceae **(Primrose family)**

Common Names:
Common Rock Jasmine

Description:
Common Rock Jasmine is a perennial herb. Leaf rosettes solitary or several forming lax mats, 3-5 cm in diameter - slightly hairy leaves. Umbels of pink flowers with yellow eyes in late spring. It is in flower from July to August. The flowers are hermaphrodite (has both male and female organs) The plant prefers light (sandy) and medium (loamy) soils, requires well-drained soil and can grow in nutritionally poor soil. This flower is native to the Himalayas, from Sikkim to Kashmir.

Medicinal Uses:
The entire plant is used in Tibetan medicine, it is said to have a bitter taste and a cooling and coarsening potency. A resolutive, it dries up serous fluids. It is used in the treatment of disorders from tumours, inflammations of fluids and other serous fluid disorders.

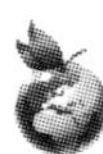

Traveller`s Joy

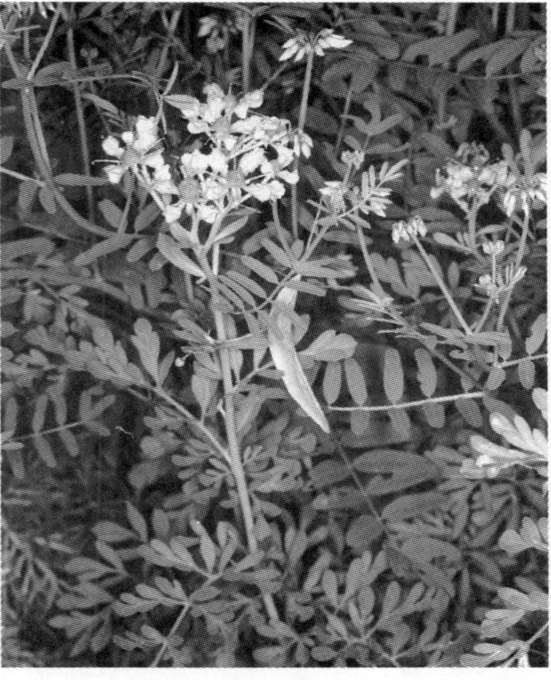

Botanical Name:

Clematis wightiana

Family:

Ranunculaceae
(Buttercup family)

Synonyms:

Clematis brachiata

Common Names:

Travellers Joy • ***Marathi:*** *Son-Jai*

Description:

Travelers Joy is a *perennial climber*, over bushes, and often simply trailing in the grass. The stems are hairy when young, but become fluted and wiry when old. The leaves are compound and opposite.

The plant climbs by means of its petioles, which on coming in contact with some support, soon make one or two coils around it. The inflorencences are shorter than the leaves.

The sweetly-scented flowers are borne in great profusion and present a common sight in autumn, along the roadsides.

The colour of the flowers range from cream-coloured to white; they are without any petals, but have four crown-shaped sepals with a powderbrush of stamens.

The seeds are greenish brown in colour and each bears a persistent feathery style, by means of which it is wind-dispersed.

The masses of fruit of the Travellers Joy are feathery in appearance. Flowering: January-April.

Medicinal Uses:

The name 'Traveller's Joy' must have come about because of all its *wonderful medicinal properties* that were useful to the traveller in days gone by when they stuffed the leaves into their shoes to ease *blisters, aches and pains.*

It's still used to *soothe muscles,* by boiling up a *strong brew from the leaves* and adding it to your *bath water.*

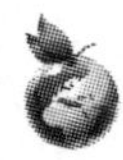

Jackal Jujube

Botanical Name:
Ziziphus oenoplia

Family:
Rhamnaceae (Ber family)

Common Names:
Jackal Jujube, Small-Fruited Jujube, Wild Jujube • Hindi: *Makkay, Makai* • Marathi: *Burgi* • Tamil: *Suraimullu, Surai ilantai* • Malayalam: *Tutali, Cheriyalanta, Tutari* • Telugu: *Paraki, Paragi, Paringi* • Kannada: *Pargi, Barige, karisurimullu, Harasurali* • Bengali: *Siakul* • Sanskrit: *Karkandhauh*

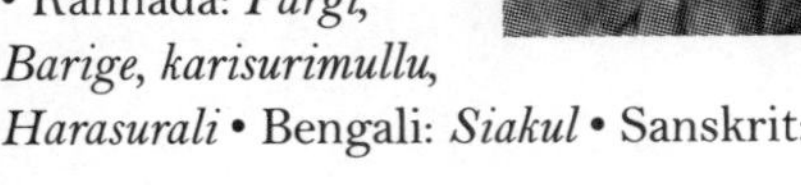

Description:
The *Jackal Jujube* is a very *thorny straggling shrub* with rusty-velvety young branches with paired thorns.

Thorns are one straight and the other recurved. Alternately arranged simple leaves are ovate to ovate-lancelike, often oblique, with three prominent nerves and numerous transverse nervules.

Tiny green flowers are borne in nearly stalkless velvety cymes in leaf axils. Fruits are spherical or obovoid drupes, black, shining, seeds woody.

Medicinal Uses:

The roots are astringent *bitter*, ***anthelmintic***, ***digestive*** and ***antiseptic***. They are useful in *hyperacidity ascaris* ***infection***, ***stomachalgia*** and ***healing of*** and *wounds*.

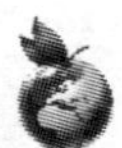

Hairy Agrimony

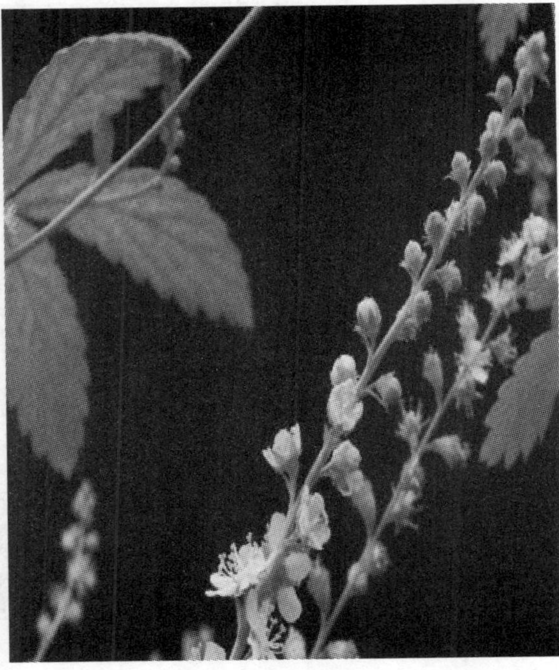

Botanical Name:

Agrimonia pilosa

Family:

Rosaceae **(Rose family)**

Synonyms:

Agrimonia dahurica

Common Names:

Hairy Agrimony, Downy agrimony
• Nepali: *Bherakuro*

Description:

Hairy Agrimony is a hairy perennial herb with erect unbranched stem 1-5 ft high. Leaves are pinnate and hairy. Leaflets are elliptic-lancelike, coarsely blunt-toothed, increasing in size from base to above. Stipules (tiny leaf-like objects at the base of leaves) are large, leafy and toothed. Tiny yellow, 5-petalled flowers, 5 mm across, are borne on a long slender spike-like cluster. Sepal cup is grooved, topped with bristles - sepals triangular. Petals are oblong-obovate. fruit is top-shaped, with ring of hooked bristles above. Hairy Agrimony is found in the Himalayas at altitudes of 1000-3000 m. Flowering: June-September.

Medicinal Uses:

The plant is used in the *treatment of abdominal pain, sore throats, headaches, bloody and mucoid dysentery, bloody and white discharge* and heat-strokes.

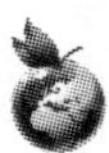

Yellow Himalayan Raspberry

Botanical Name:

Rubus ellipticus

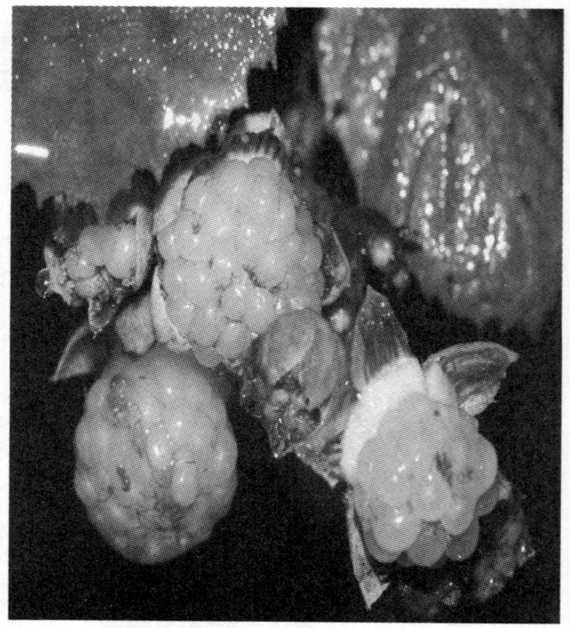

Family:

Rosaceae **(Rose family)**

Synonyms:

Rubus rotundifolius

Common Names:

Yellow Himalayan Raspberry • Hindi: *Lalanchu, Hinsal* • Manipuri: *Heijampet* • Mao: *Shingu shi* • Kashmiri: *Gouriphal, Hisara* • Assamese: *Jotelupoka* • Gujarati: *Shunu mukram* • Nepali: *Ainselu*

Description:

Yellow Himalayan Raspberry is a shrub, growing up to 2 m tall. It is clothed with prickles and reddish hairs. The alternate leaves are compound with three round to blunt leaflets 5-10 cm long.

The undersides of the leaves are lighter than the upper surface and covered with downy hairs. The flowers are small, white with five petals.

The fruit is a round yellow cluster of druplets easily detaching from the receptacle. The prickly shrub invades native forests principally in pig-disturbed habitats.

The plant has underground shoots that contribute to its spread and allow it to rapidly regenerate following a fire. The fruits are edible and frugivorous birds spread the seeds.

The Himalayan raspberry can invade disturbed habitats and displace other plant species. Yellow Himalayan Raspberry is native to India and south Asia. Flowering: February-April.

Medicinal Uses:

In Meghalaya, the *root* mixed with the *dried fruit* of *Brucea javanica* are given in *dysentery.*

Gummy Gardenia

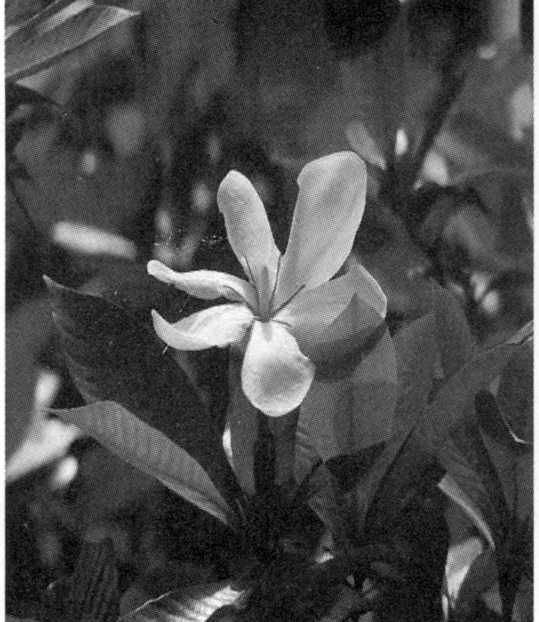

Botanical Name:

Gardenia gummifera

Family:

Rubiaceae **(Coffee family)**

Common Names:

Gummy gardenia, Cambi gum tree • Hindi: *Dekamali* • Kannada: *Kad Bikke* • Tamil: *Sịrukkambil* • Telugu: *Cittamali* • Gujarati: *Dikamalli* • Malayalam: *Kambimaram* • Sanskrit: *Nadihingu* • Marathi: *Dikemali*

Description:

Native to India, Gummy gardenia is a small tree which grows up to 3 meters. Gardenia is a genus of about 250 species of flowering plants. They are evergreen shrubs and small trees growing to 1-15 m tall. The leaves are opposite or in whorls of three or four, 5-50 cm long and 3-25 cm broad, dark green and glossy with a leathery texture. The flowers are solitary or in small clusters, white or pale yellow, with a tubular-based corolla with 5-12 lobes ('petals') from 5-12 cm diameter.

Medicinal Uses:

This species can be helpful in *treating digestive problems*, including *dyspepsia* and *diarrhoea*; or used as an *astringent* and *expectorant* for *nervous conditions* and *spasms.*

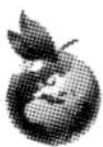

Great Morinda

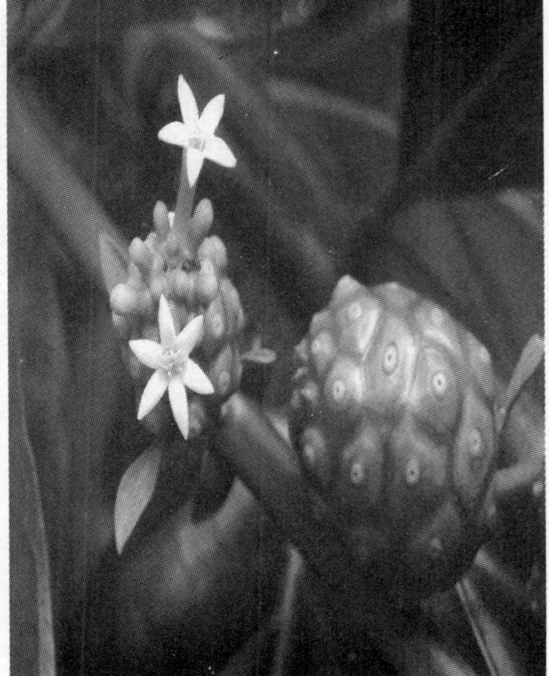

Botanical Name:

Morinda citrifolia

Family:

Rubiaceae **(Coffee family)**

Common Names:

Indian Mulberry, Great morinda • Hindi: *Bartundi* • Telugu: *Mogali* • Marathi: *Nagakunda* • Tamil: *Nuna* • Malayalam: *Mannapavatta* • Kannada: *Tagase maddi* • Gujarati: *Surangi* • Oriya: *Pindre* • Bengali: *Hurdi* • Konkani: *Bartondi*

Description:

Great morinda is a shrub or small tree native to Southeast Asia but has been extensively spread by man throughout India and into the Pacific islands as far as the islands of French Polynesian, of which Tahiti is the most prominent. It can also be found in parts of the West Indies.

The plant grows well on sandy or rocky shores. Apart from saline conditions, the plant also can withstand drought and grows in secondary soils.

It can grow up to 9 m tall, and has large, simple, dark green, shiny and deeply veined leaves. The plant flowers and fruits all year round. The flowers are small and white.

The fruit is a multiple fruit that has a pungent odour when ripening, and is hence also known as cheese fruit or even vomit fruit. It is oval and reaches 4-7 cm in size.

At first green, the fruit turns yellow then almost white as it ripens. It contains many seeds.

It is sometimes called starvation fruit. Despite its strong smell and bitter taste, the fruit is nevertheless eaten as a famine food.

Medicinal Uses:

Scientific studies have investigated the effect of this medicinal plant on the growth of cancerous *tissues.*

One such study found that this plant inhibited and reduced the *growth of the capillary vessels* sprouting from the *human breast tumour* explants and at increased concentrations, it caused existing vessels to rapidly degenerate.

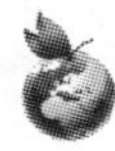

Indian Pavetta

Botanical Name:
Pavetta indica

Family:
Rubiaceae **(Coffee family)**

Synonyms:
Pavetta crassicaulis

Common Names:
Indian Pavetta, Indian Pellet Shrub • Hindi: *Kankara, Kathachampa* • Manipuri: *Kukurchura* • Marathi: *Papat* • Tamil: *Kattukkaranai,* Karanai • Malayalam: *Mallikamutti* • Telugu: *Papidi* • Kannada: *Pavati* • Bengali: *Jui* • Oriya: *Paniphingi* • Assamese: *Sam-suku* • Sanskrit: *Kakachdi*

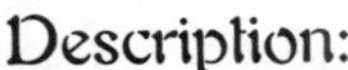

Description:
The *Indian Pavetta* is an erect, nearly smooth or somewhat hairy shrub 2 to 4 meters or more in height.

The leaves are elliptic-oblong to elliptic-lanceolate, 6-15 cm long, and pointed at both ends. The flowers are white, rather fragrant, and borne in considerable numbers in hairy terminal panicles which are 6-10 cm long. The sepals are very small, and toothed.

The flower-tube is slender and about 1.5 cm long, with obtuse petals about half the length of the tube.

The flowers attract butterflies and insects. The fruit is black when dry, somewhat rounded, and about 6 mm in diameter.

Medicinal Uses:

The *bark*, in decoction, or pulverised, is administered, especially to children, to correct *visceral obstructions.* The decocted leaves are used externally to alleviate the pains caused by *haemorrhoids.*

The *root*, pulverised and mixed with ginger and rice-water, is given in *dropsy.* A local fomentation with the *leaves* is useful in relieving the pain of piles.

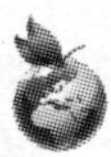

Curry Leaf

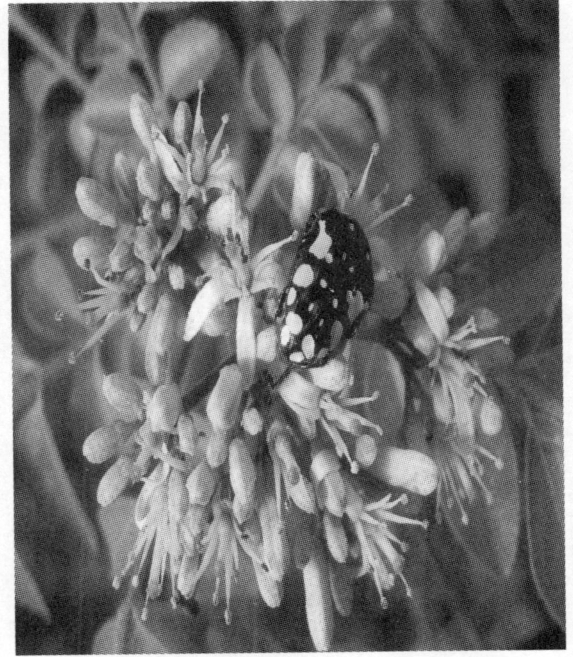

Botanical Name:
Bergera koenigii

Family:
Rutaceae **(Citrus family)**

Synonyms:
Murraya koenigii, Chalcas koenigii

Common Names:
Curry Leaf • Hindi: *Kari patta* • Marathi: *Kudianim* • Tamil: *Karivepillai* • Malayalam: *Kareapela* • Telugu: *Karepaku, Karepeku, Kari-vepa-chettu* • Kannada: *Gandhabevu, Kari-bevinagida* • Bengali: *Barsunga* • Oriya: *Lesunadando* • Assamese: *Bishahari, Narasingha* • Mizo: *Arpatil* • Sanskrit: *Alakavhaya, Chhardighna, Girinimba, Kadarya*

Description:
Curry Leaf tree is a small or medium sized tree, most famous for its aromatic leaves that provide curry spice. Curry leaves are extensively used in Southern India and Sri Lanka (and are absolutely necessary for the authentic flavour), but are also of some importance in Northern India.

It is a small tree, growing 4-6 m tall, with a trunk up to 40 cm diameter. The leaves are pinnate, with 11-21 leaflets, each leaflet 2-4 cm long and 1-2 cm broad. They are highly aromatic.

The flowers are small white, and fragrant. The small black, shiny berries are edible, but their seeds are poisonous.

Together with South Indian immigrants, curry leaves reached Malaysia, South Africa and Réunion island. When cooking, the leaves are generally used fresh off of the tree.

Outside the Indian sphere of influence, they are rarely found. The yellow "curry powder" that is common in Western countries is actually not curry at all, but a mix of spices intended to mimic the true curry flavour.

The yellow colour comes from turmeric root.

Medicinal Uses:

Leaves are *digestive, tonic, stimulant, rich in vitamin A* and *calcium.* Leaves are also used for *diarrhoea, dysentry* and *checking vomitting. Bark-paste* is antisceptic, applied to skin eruptions.

Root extract is taken for *relief* from *renal pain.*

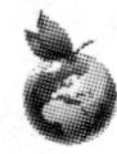

Ceylon Satinwood

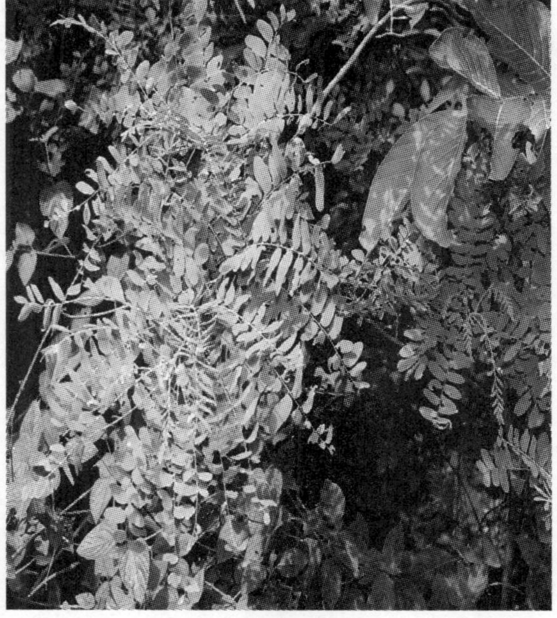

Botanical Name:
Chloroxylon swietenia

Family:
Rutaceae **(Citrus family)**

Synonyms:
Swietenia chloroxylon

Common Names:
Ceylon Satinwood, East Indian Satinwood, Buruta • Hindi: *Bhirra, Bhivia, Dhoura, Girya* • Marathi: *Behru, Halda, Bheria, Hulda* • Tamil: *Vaaimaram or Porasu, Mammarai, Porinja maram* • Malayalam: *Varimaram* • Telugu: *Billu, Billydu, Billudu, Bella* • Kannada: *Bittulla, Huragalu, Hurihuli, Masula* • Oriya: *Bheru gatcho* • Sanskrit: *Bhillotaka, Bimbilota*

Description:
Ceylon Satinwood is a hardwood tree, native to south India and Sri Lanka. Ceylon Satinwood is a medium-sized deciduous tree, growing to 15-20 m tall, with thick, fissured, slightly corky bark.

Alternately arranged leaves are 15-22 cm long, pinnately divided into 10-20 pairs of oblong, blunt leaflets. The flowers are small, creamy-white, produced in panicles 10-20 cm long.

Buds are round. the fruit is an oblong three-segmented capsule 2.5-4.5 cm long, containing 1-4 seeds in each segment.

The wood produced by the tree is often a golden colour with a reflective sheen. It is used for small luxury items and as a veneer in wooden furniture. It is one of the best-known satinwoods.

Medicinal Uses:

Ceylon Satinwood is used in *folk medicine* in *Chhattisgarh*. In case of a *problematic wound*, the *dried leaves* of Ceylon Satinwood are applied on the wound in order to increase the healing process.

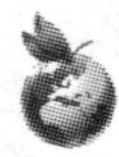

Lavang Lata

Botanical Name:
Luvunga scandens

Family:
Rutaceae **(Citrus family)**

Synonyms:
Limonia scandens

Common Names:
Lavang Lata, Indian lavanga
• Hindi: *Lavang lata*
• Manipuri: *Lavang Lata* • Kannada: *Jeeanthi balli, Jeevani, Kakkola, Lavangalathe*
• Bengali: *Lavang Lata*
• Assamese: *Lavang Lata* • Sanskrit:
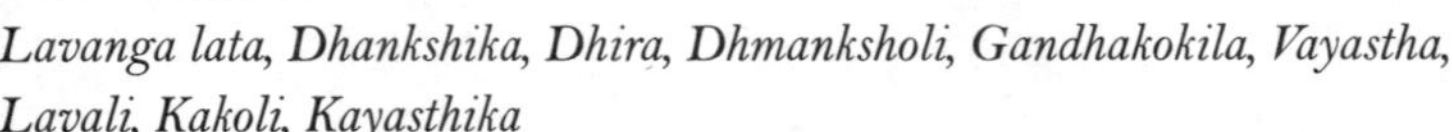
Lavanga lata, Dhankshika, Dhira, Dhmanksholi, Gandhakokila, Vayastha, Lavali, Kakoli, Kayasthika

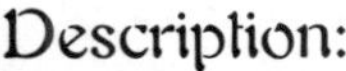

Description:
Lavang Lata is a strong woody climber with recurved spines, native to North-East India. It belongs to the family of lemon and orange. Unfortunately, it has now become a rare and endangered species.

Leaves are compound, with 3 leaflets which are lancelike and leathery. Leaf stalks are chanelled. Peduncles carrying 4-12 pretty large, white, fragrant flowers, arise from leaf axils.

Flowers are shaped like the flowers of most citrus plants. Fruit is oblong, 2.5 x 2 cm in size, yellowish, with smooth aromatic peel and resinous, fragrant pulp. The fruit has 1-3 ovoid seeds. This evergreen plant is sometimes grown for ornamental purposes. Flowering: March-April.

Medicinal Uses:

Dried fruits are used in making *medicinal oil. Roots* and *fruits* are employed for treating *scorpion-stings.*

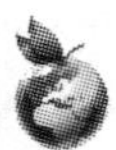

Rue

Botanical Name:

Ruta graveolens

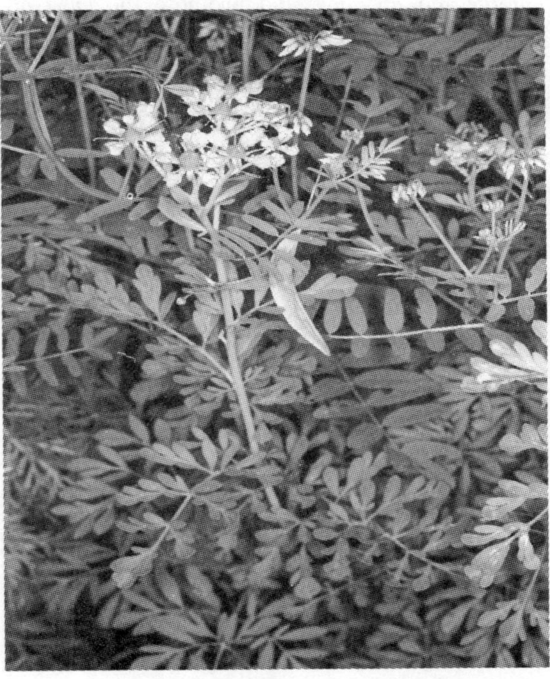

Family:

Rutaceae **(Citrus family)**

Common Names:

Rue, Common rue, herb of Grace • Hindi: *Sadab, Saturi* • Marathi: *Satapa* • *Tamil: Aruvadam* • Malayalam: *Sadsu* • Telugu: *Sadapa* • Kannada: *Satari* • Bengali: *Ispund* • Oriya: *Maruya* • Sanskrit: *Sarpadanshta*

Description:

Rue is a small evergreen subshrub or semiwoody perennial 2-3 ft tall and almost as wide. It is sometimes grown as an ornamental plant in gardens, especially because of its bluish leaves, and also sometimes for its tolerance of hot and dry soil conditions.

It also is grown as both a medicinal herb and as a condiment. The 3-5 in long leaves are dissected pinnately into oblong or spoon shaped segments.

They are somewhat fleshy and usually covered with a powdery bloom. The sea green foliage has a strong, pungent, rather unpleasant scent when bruised.

The paniculate clusters of small yellow flowers appear in spring, held well above the foliage and often covering most of the plant. Each flower is about 0.5 in across with four concave notched petals.

Rue usually grows in a compact, rounded mound. Common rue is native to southern Europe and northern Africa.

Medicinal Uses:

In *European folk medicine*, Rue is said to relieve *gas pains* and *colic*, *improve appetite* and *digestion*, and promote the *onset of menstruation* and *uteral contractions*.

For this reason the refined oil of rue has been cited by the Roman historian Pliny the Elder and the gynecologist Soranus, as a potent abortifacient (inducing abortion).

Rue contains pilocarpine which is used in horses to *induce abortion*, and is a traditional abortifacient among Hispanic people in New Mexico.

Winged Prickly Ash

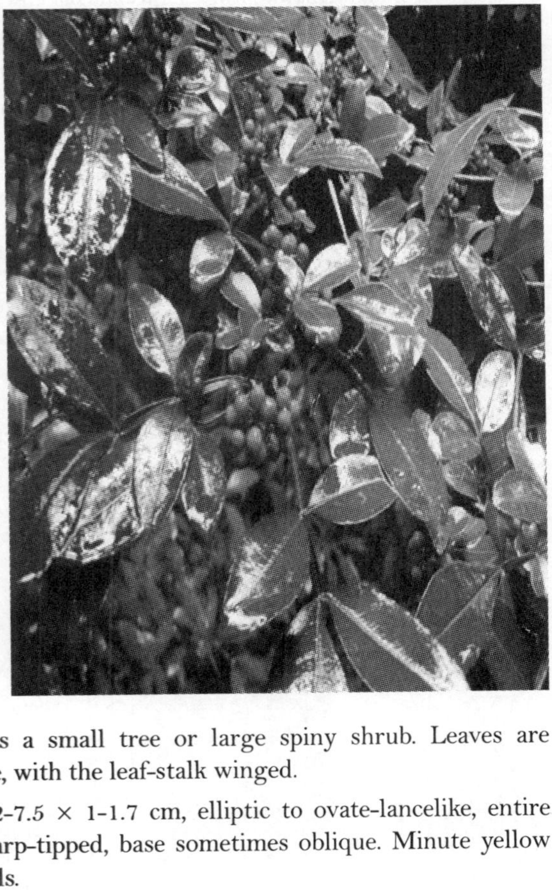

Botanical Name:
Zanthoxylum armatum

Family:
Rutaceae **(Citrus family)**

Synonyms:
Zanthoxylum alatum

Common Names:
Winged Prickly Ash, Prickly ash, Tumbru, Toothache Tree, Tejbal, Yellow wood, Suterberry • Hindi: *Tejphal, Darmar*
• Manipuri: ***Mukthrubi***
• Tamil: ***Timur***
• Telugu: ***Konda-Kasimi***
• Kannada: ***Jimmi***

Description:
Winged Prickly Ash is a small tree or large spiny shrub. Leaves are distinctlively trifoliolate, with the leaf-stalk winged.

Leaflets are stalkless, 2-7.5 × 1-1.7 cm, elliptic to ovate-lancelike, entire to slightly toothed, sharp-tipped, base sometimes oblique. Minute yellow flowers arise in leaf axils.

Flowers have 6-8 acute sepals. Petals are absent. Male flowers have 6-8 stamens, and large anthers because of which the flowers look yellow.

Female flowers have 1-3 celled ovary, 3 mm in diameter, pale red, splitting into two when ripe.

Seed are rounded, 3 mm in diameter, shining black. Flowering: March-April.

Medicinal Uses:

Prickly Ash is used in *many chronic problems* such as *rheumatism* and *skin diseases,* cramps in the legs varicose veins and varicose ulcers.

It is also used for *low blood pressure, fever* and *inflammation.* Externally, it may be used as a *stimulation liniment* for *rheumatism* and *fibrositis.*

It has a stimulating effect upon the *lymphatic system, circulation* and *mucous membranes.*

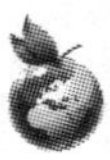

Indian Willow

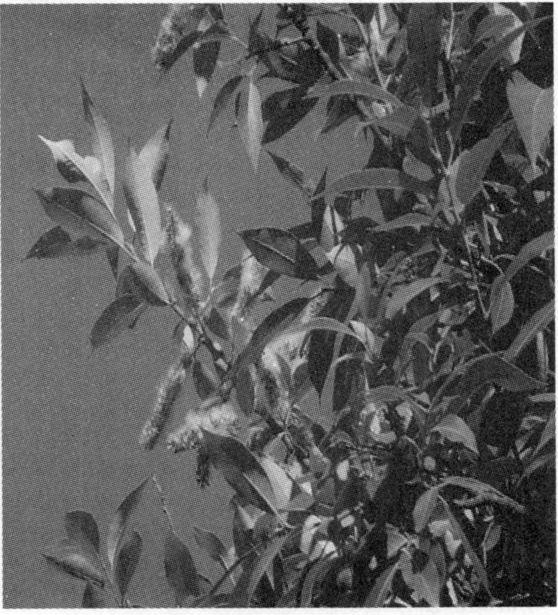

Botanical Name:

Salix tetrasperma

Family:

Salicaceae **(Willow family)**

Common Names:

Indian Willow

- Hindi: *Bod, Bains*
- Manipuri: *Ooyum*
- Bengali: *Panijama*
- Tamil: *Atrupalai*
- Kannada: *Niranji*
- Malayalam: *Arali, Atrupala*

Description:

The Indian Willow is a *medium sized tree* of *wet and swampy places,* shedding the leaves at the end of monsoon. It flowers after leafing. The bark is rough, with deep, vertical fissures. The young shoots and young leaves are silky. The leaves are lance-like, or ovate-lancelike, 8-15 cm long, with minutely and regularly toothed margins. The male sweet scented catkins are 5-10 cm long, and are borne on leafy branchlets. The female catkins are 8-12 cms long. The capsules are long, stipulate, in groups of 3 to 4. In Manipur, in NE India, the new flowers of Indian Willow, locally known as (Ooyum), lightly boiled and mixed with mashed boiled potatoes, and are considered delcicious. Flowering: January-February.

Medicinal Uses:

The *bark of The Indian Willow* is used to *treat fever.*

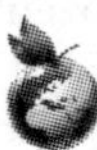

Mahua

Botanical Name:
Madhuca longifolia var. latifolia

Family:
Sapotaceae **(Mahua family)**

Synonyms:
Bassia latifolia, Illipe latifolia, Madhuca indica, Madhuca latifolia

Common Names:
Indian Butter Tree
• Hindi: *Mahua*
• Bengali: *Maul*
• Hindi: *Mohwa*
• Marathi: *Kat-illipi*
• Malayalam: *Illupa* • Telugu: *Ippa*

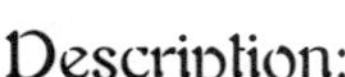

Description:
Mohwa is one of the most important of Indian forest trees, not because it may possess valuable timber - and it is hardly ever cut for this purpose - but because of its delicious and nutritive flowers.

It is a tree of abundant growth and, to the people of Central India, it provides their most important article of food as the flowers can be stored almost indefinitely.

It is large and deciduous with a thick, grey bark, vertically cracked and wrinkled. Most of the leaves fall from February to April, and during that time the musky-scented flowers appear.

They hang in close bunches of a dozen or so from the end of the gnarled, grey branchlets.

Actually the word 'hang' is incorrect because, when a bunch is inverted, the flower stalks are sufficiently rigid to maintain their position. These stalks are green or pink and furry, about 5 cm. long.

The plum-coloured calyx is also furry and divides into four or five lobes; within them lies the globular corolla, thick, juicy and creamy white. Through small eyelet holes at the top, the yellow anthers can be seen.

The stamens are very short and adhere to the inner surface of the corolla; the pistil is a long, protruding green tongue. It is at night that the tree blooms and at dawn each short-lived flower falls to the ground.

A couple of months after the flowering period the fruit opens. They are fleshy, green berries, quite large and containing from one to four shiny, brown seeds.

Medicinal Uses:

Medicinally, the tree is very valuable. The *bark* is used to *cure leprosy* and to *heal wounds*, the *flowers* are prepared to *relieve coughs*, *biliousness* and *heart-trouble*, while the *fruit* is given in cases of *consumption* and *blood diseases.*

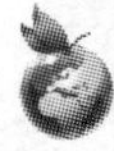

South Indian Mahua

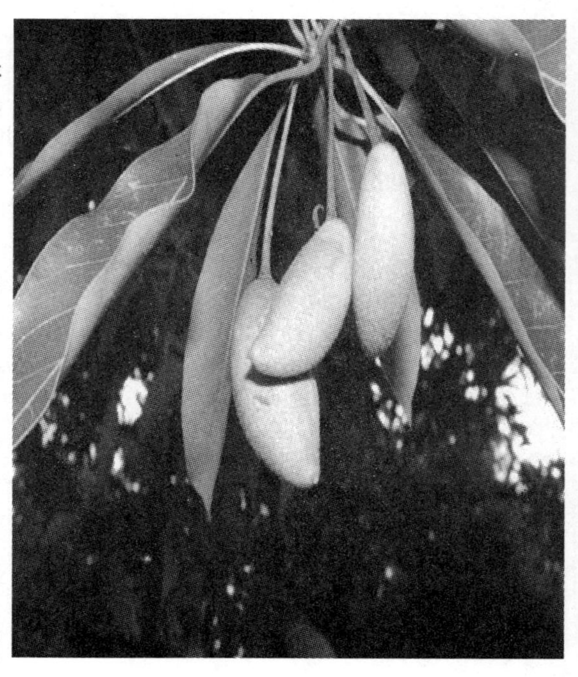

Botanical Name:

Madhuca longifolia var. longifolia

Family:

Sapotaceae (**Mahua family**)

Common Names:

South Indian Mahua, Indian Butter Tree

- Hindi: *Mahua*
- Bengali: *Maul*
- Marathi: *Mohwa*
- Tamil: *Kat-illipi*
- Malayalam: *Illupa*
- Telugu: *Ippa*

Description:

The South Indian Mahua is a variety of Mahua which is predominently found in South India. It differs from the usual Mahua in that its leaves are narrower.

Mohua is one of the most important of Indian forest trees, not because it may possess valuable timber - and it is hardly ever cut for this purpose - but because of its delicious and nutritive flowers.

It is a tree of abundant growth and, to the people of Central India, it provides their most important article of food as the flowers can be stored almost indefinitely.

It is large and deciduous with a thick, grey bark, vertically cracked and wrinkled. Most of the leaves fall from February to April, and during that time the musky-scented flowers appear.

They hang in close bunches of a dozen or so from the end of the gnarled, grey branchlets.

The reddish young leaves with the flower clusters look very attractive. The flower stalks are green or pink and furry, about 5 cm. long. The plum-coloured calyx is also furry and divides into four or five lobes; within them lies the globular corolla, thick, juicy and creamy white.

Through small eyelet holes at the top, the yellow anthers can be seen. The stamens are very short and adhere to the inner surface of the corolla; the pistil is a long, protruding green tongue.

It is at night that the tree blooms and at dawn each short-lived flower falls to the ground. A couple of months after the flowering period the fruit opens.

They are fleshy, green berries, quite large and containing from one to four shiny, brown seeds.

Medicinal Uses:

Medicinally, the tree is very valuable. The *bark* is used to *cure leprosy* and to *heal wounds*, the *flowers* are prepared to *relieve coughs*, *biliousness* and *heart-trouble*, while the fruit is given in cases of *consumption* and *blood diseases.*

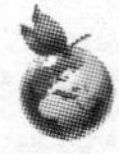

Maulsari

Botanical Name:

Mimusops elengi

Family:

Sapotaceae (**Mahua family**)

Common Names:

Spanish cherry

- Hindi: *Maulsari*
- Urdu: *Kirakuli*
- Manipuri: *Bokul lei*
- Tamil: *Magizhamboo*
- Malayalam: *Ilanni*
- Bengali: *Bakul*
- Marathi: *Bakuli*
- Konkani: *Omval*
- Kannada: *Ranjal*
- Gujarati: *Barsoli*

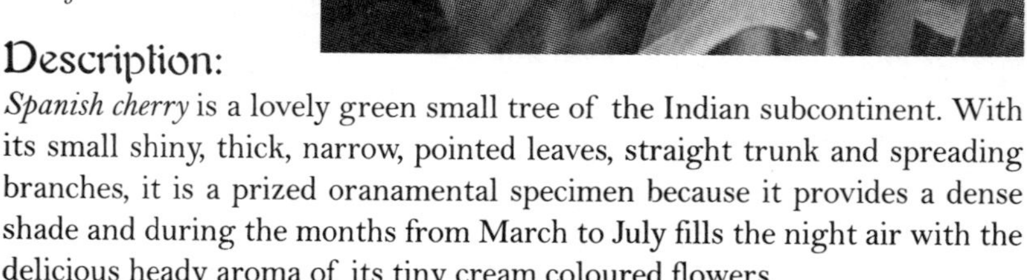

Description:

Spanish cherry is a lovely green small tree of the Indian subcontinent. With its small shiny, thick, narrow, pointed leaves, straight trunk and spreading branches, it is a prized oranamental specimen because it provides a dense shade and during the months from March to July fills the night air with the delicious heady aroma of its tiny cream coloured flowers.

Flowers are small, star-shaped, yellowish white in colour, with a crown rising from the centre. Oval leaves, wavy at margin, about 5-16 cm and 3-7 cm wide.

In the morning, the fragrant flowers which so graciously scented their surroundings with their deep, rich, fragrance during the evening hours, fall to the ground.

People love to collect them as they retain their odour for many days after they fall.

They are offered in temples and shrines throughout the country. Appears in Indian mythology as *Vakula* - said to put forth blossoms when sprinkled with nectar from the mouth of lovely women. Fruits are eaten fresh.

Medicinal Uses:

Various parts of the tree have medicinal properties. It is used in the *treatment and maintenance of oral hygiene.*

Rinsing mouth with water solution made with *bakul* helps in *strengthening the teeth.* It also *prevents bad breath* and helps *keep the gums healthy.*

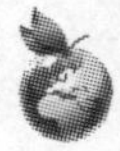

Chameleon Plant

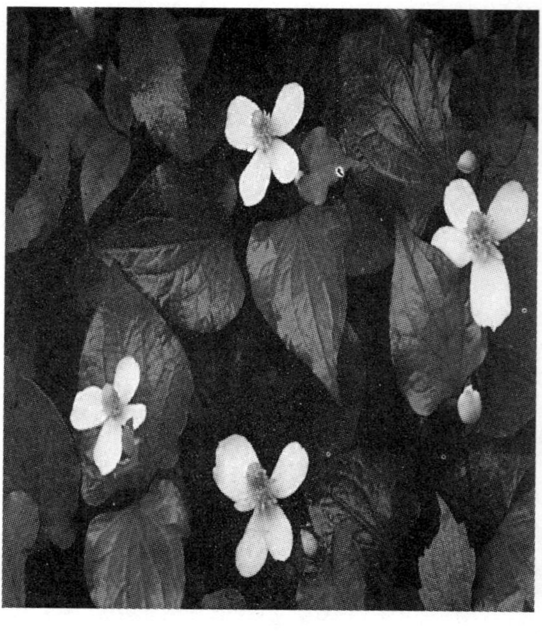

Botanical Name:

Houttuynia cordata

Family:

Saururaceae **(lizard-tail family)**

Common Names:

Chameleon Plant • Manipuri: *Toningkhok*

Description:

The Chameleon Plant is a perennial ground cover plant. It is been marketed as a creeping ornamental garden plant, which has heart shaped leaves up to 75 mm long and almost as wide. The leaves are comprised of a mixture of colours from green through yellow to red, the brighter colours being more prominent when grown in full sunlight. The leaves are opposite along thin erect stems which arise from slender rhizomes. The minute flowers are densely clustered on short spikes. At the base of each spike are four white petal-like parts. The leaves of Chameleon Plant are heart-shaped, usually green, but take on various colours like variegated cream, bronze, scarlet, and have a peppery scent when crushed. The leaves make a marvelous flavouring in salads. In Manipur, people love it and consume it in various ways, as salad, also in *pakodas.*

Medicinal Uses:

The *Leaf-extract* is used in *dysentry* and the rhizome is used in *stomach ulcers.* Boiled *extract of the rhizomes* is taken for *muscular pains* due to *overstrain.*

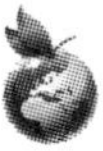

Brahmi

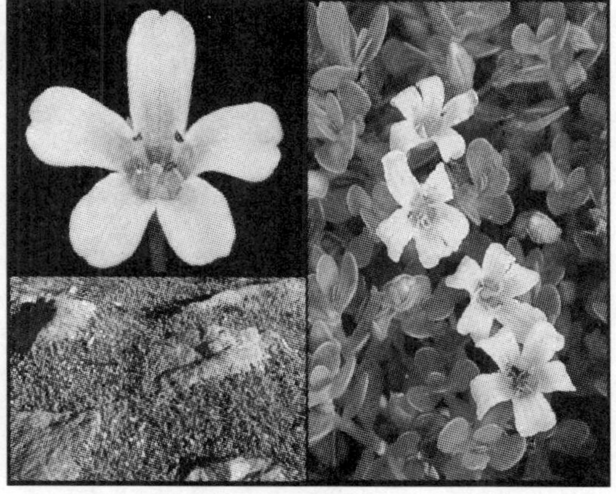

Botanical Name:
Bacopa monnieri

Family:
Scrophulariaceae **(Dog flower family)**

Common Names:
Water Hyssop, Indian pennywort • Hindi: *Brahmi* • Tamil: *Nirbrahmi* • Gujarati: *Jalanevari*

Description:
Brahmi is a perennial, creeping herb whose habitat includes wetlands and muddy shores. The leaves of this plant are succulent and relatively thick.

Leaves are oblanceolate and are arranged oppositely on the stem. The flowers are small and white, with four or five petals. Its ability to grow in water makes it a popular aquarium plant.

It can even grow in slightly brackish conditions. Propagation is often achieved through cuttings.

It commonly grows in marshy areas throughout India, Nepal, Sri Lanka, China, Taiwan, and is also found in Florida and other southern states where it can be grown in damp conditions by the pond or bog garden.

Medicinal Uses:
Famed in *Ayurvedic medicine,* the Brahmi has *antioxidant properties.* It has been reported to *reduce the oxidation of fats in the blood stream,* which is a risk factor for *cardiovascular diseases.*

It has been used for centuries to help benefit *epilepsy, memory capacity,* increase concentration, and reduce stress-induced anxiety.

According to *Ayurveda,* it's bitter, pungent, heating, emetic, *laxative* and useful in *bad ulcers, tumours, ascites, enlargement of the spleen, indigestion, inflammations, leprosy, anaemia, biliousness* etc.

According to the *Unani system of medicine,* it's *bitter, aphrodisiac,* good in *scabies, leucoderma, syphilis,* etc. It is a promising blood purifier and useful in diarrhoea and fevers.

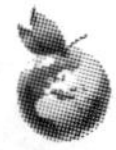

Horned Lousewort

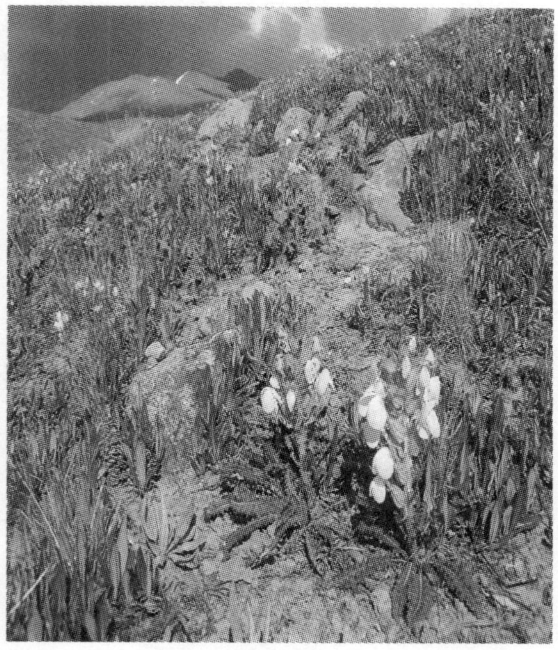

Botanical Name:

Pedicularis bicornuta

Family:

Scrophulariaceae **(Dog flower family)**

Common Names:

Horned Lousewort, Lousewort

Description:

Horned Lousewort, the curious species, inhabits tough and sometimes inaccessible areas of the Himalayan cold deserts.

The plants are tough and sturdy and the corolla of these flowers are closed in a ball-like fashion to cover the delicate vital parts such as the *stamens* and *stigma* from the outside pressures. The flowers have interesting cultural use in certain Himalayan areas.

The flowers are considered an integral offering to please Goddess Kali and get one's wishes fulfilled. Further, no religious ceremony is considered to be complete without the offering of these flowers in the first prayers.

The women also make garlands from the flowers to greet each other on important religious occasions and to garland Goddess Kali during festivals.

Horned lousewort is a robust, erect perennial which grows upto 60 cm, with dense clusters of large globular yellow flowers.

Leaves are alternately arranged, and are pinnately lobed.

Flowers are 2 cm across. The calyx (the tube consisting of sepals) is inflated and hairy.

The flower tube is narrow and hairy. The upper lip of the flower is s-shaped or spirally curved with slender two-lobed beak.

Medicinal Uses:

The *flowers* of this plant are used in *Tibetan medicine*, and they are said to have a *bitter taste* and a *cooling potency.*

They are used in the treatment of *vaginal* and *seminal discharges.*

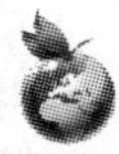

Sweet Broom Weed

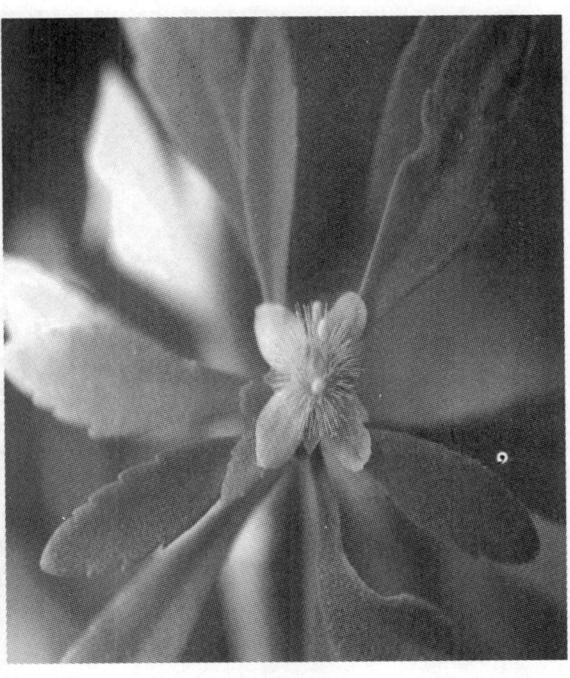

Botanical Name:
Scoparia dulcis

Family:
Scrophulariaceae **(Dog flower family)**

Common Names:
Sweet Broom Weed, Sweet Broom Wort • Hindi: *Mithi patti, Ghoda tulsi* • Tamil: *Sarakkotthini* • Bengali: *Bon dhonya*

Description:
Sweet Broom Weed is a branched herb with wiry stems, growing up to 1 m tall. Narrowly elliptic, almost stalkless leaves are arranged oppositely or in whorls of 3. Leaves are 3-4 x 1-1.5 cm wide, with serrated margins. Small white, hairy flowers occur in leaf axils. The stamens are greenish and the ovary is green. The capsule is nearly round.

Medicinal Uses:
It is traditionally used in the treatment of *diabetes, dysentery, earaches, fevers, gonorrhoea, headaches, jaundice, snake-bites, stomach problems, toothaches,* warts, etc.

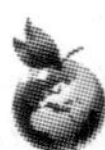

Asiatic Witchweed

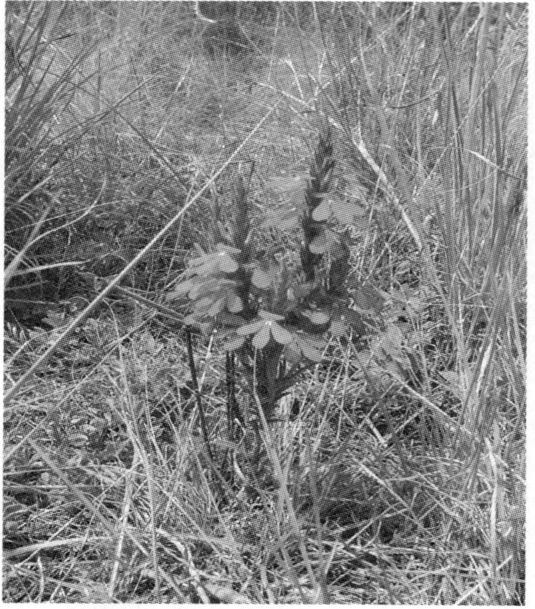

Botanical Name:
Striga asiatica

Family:
Scrophulariaceae **(Dog flower family)**

Synonyms:
Striga lutea

Common Names:
Asiatic Witchweed • Marathi: *Pivla agya* • Tamil: *Pallipoondu, Kollaippalli, Chirakachitam, Chirakacitappuntu* • Malayalam: *Kalu-polapen* • Telugu: *Rathi badamika* • Kannada: *Bili kasa, Jolada baeru maari*

Description:
Asiatic Witchweed is a coarse annual herb, growing to 10-20 cm tall. Stems are erect, rarely branched. Leaf are small, linear to narrowly lance shaped, 5-20 mm long, 1-4 mm wide, sometimes reduced to scales. Flowers arise singly or in a spike in leaf axils. Sepal cup is 4-8 mm, 10-ribbed. Sepals are 5, as long as tube. Flowers are usually yellow, rarely red or white, with a 0.8-1.5 cm long tube, and 2-lipped. Upper lip is 2-lobed. Capsule is ovoid, enveloped in surviving sepals. This species is harmful to crops, particularly to sugar cane. Flowering: September-October.

Medicinal Uses:
The *whole plant* is used for treating *intestinal parasites.*

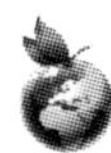

Indian Tree of Heaven

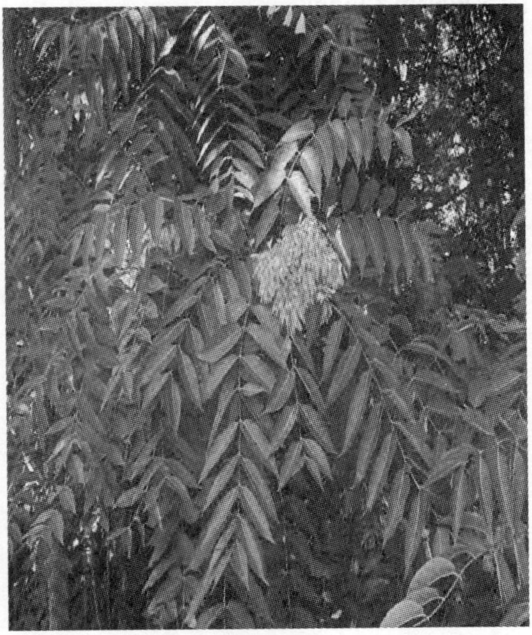

Botanical Name:
Ailanthus excelsa

Family:
Simaroubaceae **(Quassia family)**

Common Names:
Indian Tree of Heaven, Coramandel ailanto • Hindi: *Mahanimb, Maharukh* • Marathi: *Marukh, Mahrukh, Mahanimb* • Tamil: *Agal, Perumaram, Perumaruntu* • Malayalam: *Mattipongilyam, Peru, Perumaram* • Telugu: *Pedda, Peddamandu, Peddamanu* • Kannada: *Bende, Dodabevu, Dodda* • Oriya: *Mundayigatch* • Sanskrit: *Aralu, Araluka, Araluvrksa*

Description:
The Indian Tree of Heaven is a large deciduous tree, 18-25 m tall; trunk straight, 60-80 cm in diameter; bark light grey and smooth, becoming grey-brown and rough on large trees. It is aromatic and slightly bitter.

Leaves alternate, pinnately compound, large, 30-60 cm or more in length; leaflets 8-14 or more pairs, long stalked, ovate or broadly lance shaped from very unequal base, 6-10 cm long, 3-5 cm wide, often curved, long pointed, hairy gland; edges coarsely toothed and often lobed.

Flower clusters droop at leaf bases, shorter than leaves, much branched; flowers many, mostly male and female on different trees, short stalked, greenish-yellow. There are five sepals, a and five narrow petals spreading 6 mm across.

Fruit a 1-seeded samara, lance shaped, flat, pointed at ends, 5 cm long, 1 cm wide, copper red, strongly veined, twisted at the base The genus name *Ailanthus* comes from *ailanthos* (tree of heaven), the Indonesian name for *Ailanthus moluccana.* Flowering: January-March.

Medicinal Uses:

The bark is used in India as a powerful *fever-cure* and *tonic.*

The *leaves* and *bark* are popularly used as a *tonic after labour,* and the *juice of the leaves* and *fresh bark* employed by the Konkans as a *remedy for after-pains.*

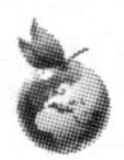

Belladonna

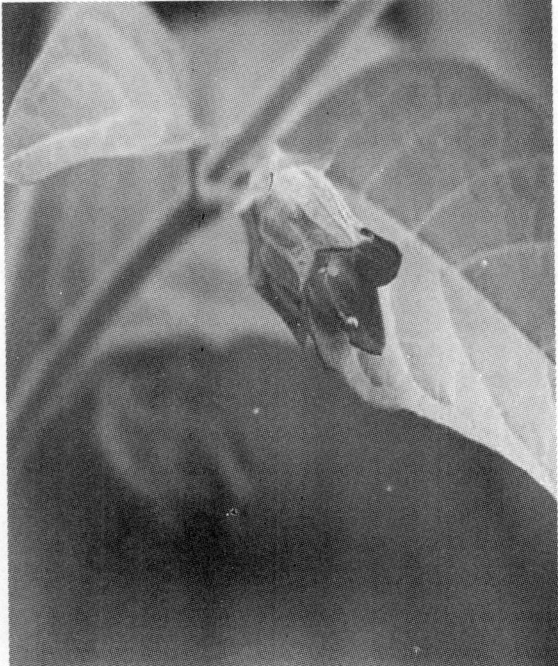

Botanical Name:
Atropa belladonna

Family:
Solanaceae **(Potato family)**

Synonyms:
Atropa bella-donna

Common Names:
Belladonna, Devil's Cherries, Naughty Man's Cherries, Divale, Black Cherry, Devil's Herb, Great Morel, Dwayberry • Hindi: *Angur Shefa, Luckmuna, Luckmunee, Sag-angur* • Tamil: *Bellatona, Pelletonacceti* • Kashmiri: *Sagangur* • Bengali: *Yebruj* • Urdu: *Bikh luffah, Poast bikh luffah* • Sanskrit: *Suchi*

Description:
Belladonna is a *perennial branching herb* growing to *5 feet tall.* The leaves are dull, darkish green in colour and of unequal size, 3-10 inches long, the lower leaves solitary, the upper ones in pairs alternately from opposite sides of the stem, one leaf of each pair much larger than the other, oval in shape, acute at the apex, entire and attenuated into short petioles.

First-year plants grow only about 1 1/2 feet in height. Their leaves are often larger than in full-grown plants and grow on the stem immediately above the ground.

Older plants attain a height of 3-5 ft, occasionally even 6 ft. The flowers, borne in leaf axils, are of a dark and dingy purplish colour, tinged with green, about 2.5 cm long, pendent, bell-shaped, furrowed.

The flowers have five large teeth or lobes, slightly reflexed. The fruit is 0.5 inch smooth berry, which ripens to acquire a shining black or purple colour.

Every part of the plant is extremely poisonous, and can result in poisoning of not handled carefully.

Medicinal Uses:

The plant is believed to be *narcotic, diuretic, sedative, antispasmodic, and mydriatic.*

Belladonna is a most valuable plant in the treatment of *eye diseases*, Atropine, obtained during extraction, being its most important constituent on account of its power of *dilating the pupil.*

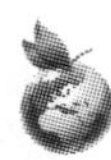

Henbane

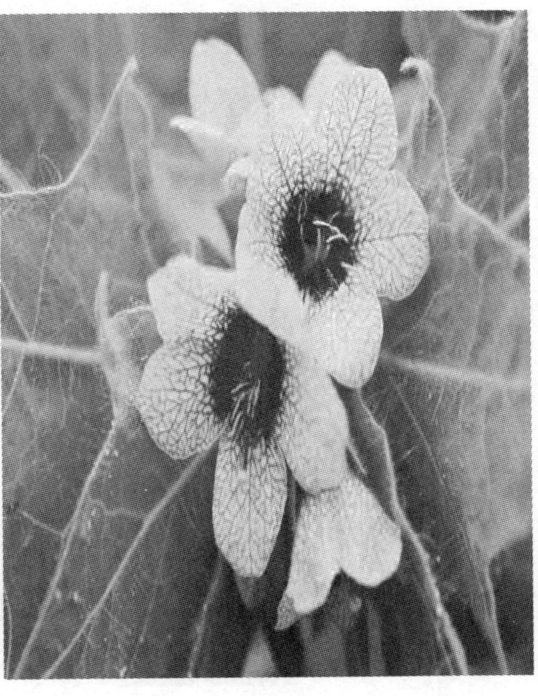

Botanical Name:

Hyoscyamus niger

Family:

Solanaceae **(Potato family)**

Common Names:

Henbane, Stinking nightshade • Hindi: *Khurasani ajwain* • Sanskrit: *Parseek yawani* • Nepali: *Khursani jwanu*

Description:

Henbane is a robust, leafy plant, growing to 1 m tall. The plant is coarsely hairy, sticky and stinks. Basal leaves are elliptic, irregularly lobed, stalked. Stem leaves are stalkless. Flowers are cup-shaped, 2-3 cm across, dull yellow, prominently netted with purple veins, and have a dark purple center. Sepal cup is funnel shaped with triangular pointed sepals. Sepals enlarge and become papery in fruit, and encircle the capsule. Henbane is found in the Himalayas at altitudes of 2100-3300 m. Flowering: May-September.

Medicinal Uses:

Henbane is used in *Homeopathic medicine.*

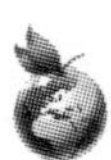

Mandrake

Botanical Name:
Mandragora officinarum

Family:
Solanaceae **(Potato family)**

Common Names:
Mandrake, Satan's Apple, Love Apple, Devil's Apple • Hindi: *Bhagener, Lakmani* • Tamil: *Katal jati, Katavjate* • Telugu: *Mantrika, Saitanu Pandu, Prema Pandu, Deyyapu Kaya* • Kannada: *Lakshmana* • Urdu: *Luffah* • Sanskrit: *Laksmana, Putrada, Raktavindu*

Description:
Mandrake is a narcotic herb, native to South-east Europe. The plant has a long tap-root that is usually split up into two parts, resembling a human form. Immediately from the crown of the root arise several large, dark-green leaves, which at first stand erect, but when grown to full size a foot or more in length and 4-5 inches in width - spread open and lie upon the ground.

They are sharp pointed at the apex and of an unpleasant odour. From among these leaves spring the flowers, each on a separate foot-stalk, 3-4 inches high.

They are somewhat of the shape and size of a primrose, the corolla bell-shaped, cut into five spreading segments, of a whitish colour, somewhat tinged with purple.

They are succeeded by a smooth, round fruit, about as large as a small apple, of a deep yellow colour when ripe, full of pulp and with a strong, apple-like scent.

In recent times, the seed of the plant was brought to South India, by some plant lovers. According to European legends, when the root is dug up it screams and kills all who hear it.

Literature includes complex directions for harvesting a mandrake root in relative safety.

Medicinal Uses:

In ancient times, it was used as *a narcotic* and an *aphrodisiac*, and it was also believed to have certain magical powers. In *large doses*, it is said to excite *delirium* and *madness*.

Mandrake was used in as an *anaesthetic for surgeries* in the *Middle Ages*, a *piece of the root* being given to the patient to chew *before undergoing the operation.* The plant is even mentioned in *Genesis*.

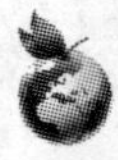

Ground Cherry

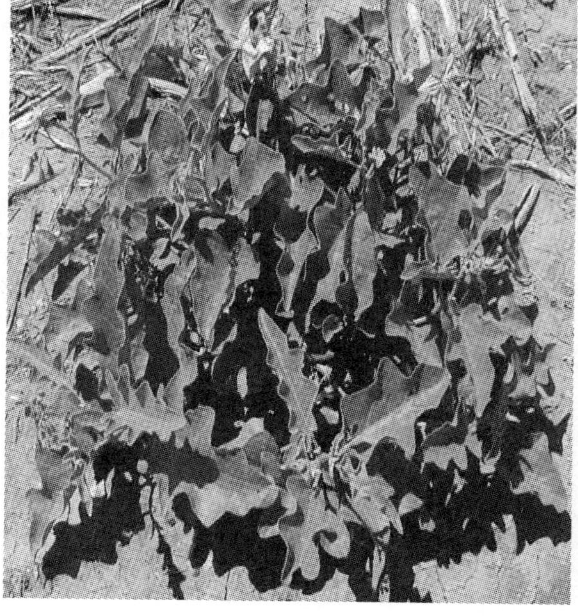

Botanical Name:

Physalis minima

Family:

Solanaceae **(Potato family)**

Common Names:

Ground Cherry, Sunberry • Hindi: *Rasbhari, Ban Tipariya, Chirpati* • Marathi: *Chirboti, Nanvachivel, Ran-popti* • Tamil: *Kupanti* • Malayalam: *Notinotta* • Telugu: *Kupanti* • Kannada: *Gadde hannu* • Bengali: *Bantepariya* • Gujarati: *Popti*

Description:

This is a popular wild fruits to pick and eat. The taste of the ripe berry is sweet and distinctive. The berries are ripe when the husk turns brown and the berry inside takes on a yellowish cast.

This is a herbaceous plant which can reach 3 ft. It can be a perennial or an annual. The stem is branched and often reclining.

The leaves are alternate. Leaves can reach 10cm in length. Each leaf is toothed or lobed.

The flowers have five (5) Regular Parts and are up to 2cm wide.

They are greenish yellow sometimes brownish yellow. Blooms first appear in early summer and continue into late summer.

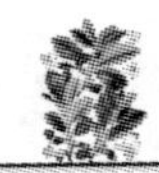

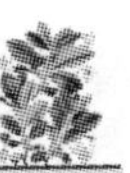

The flowers hang from the stem. A berry hidden in a larger papery shell.

The berry and shell are both green at first with the shell turning light brown and the berry taking on a yellow cast when ripe.

Medicinal Uses:

The *plant* has been used as a *diuretic* for various *urinary problems.* There seems to be no scientific data to support this.

Its use for *bladder problems* may go back to the doctrine of signatures. 'Physalis' is the Greek word for *bladder.*

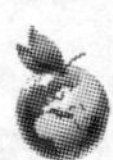

Horse Nettle

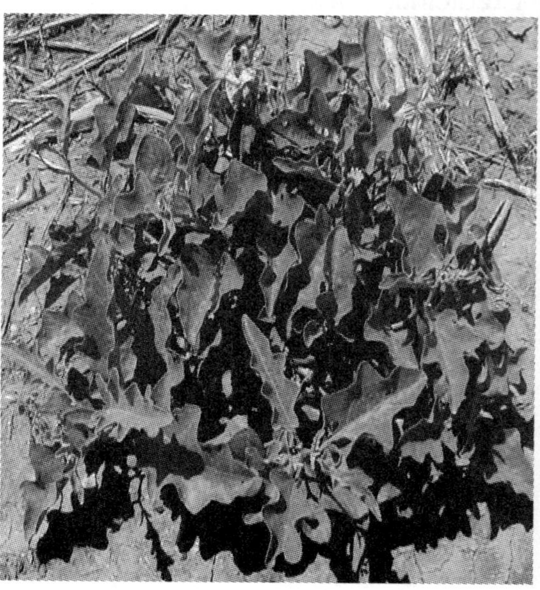

Botanical Name:

Solanum carolinense L.

Family:

Solanaceae **(Potato family)**

Common Names:

H*orse Nettle, Apple of Sodom, Carolina Horse Nettle, Nightshade*

Description:

Horse-nettle is not related to true nettles, *but rather* to *nightshade, tomatoes,* and *potatoes.* The horse nettle flower has five broad, pointed petals that form a somewhat star-shaped corolla, and the five thick stamens seem to have a "beak" shape. The thick pistil extends beyond the corolla and the stamens. Its leaves and stems are prickly. It is, however, very prickly, and though its flowers are beautiful, it is usually considered a weed. Its low status is a result of its almost unbelievable ability to stand up to attempts to eradicate it. As a result, it is frequently to be found in both cow pastures and cultivated fields, as well as in woods and meadows.

Medicinal Uses:

This plant is *extremely poisonous.* The *berries,* when properly prepared, have been used as *diuretics, antispasmodics, anodynes,* and according to the U.S. Dispensatory, they have also been used in the *treatment of epilepsy.*

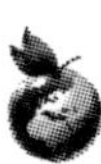

Indian Nightshade

Botanical Name:
Solanum indicum

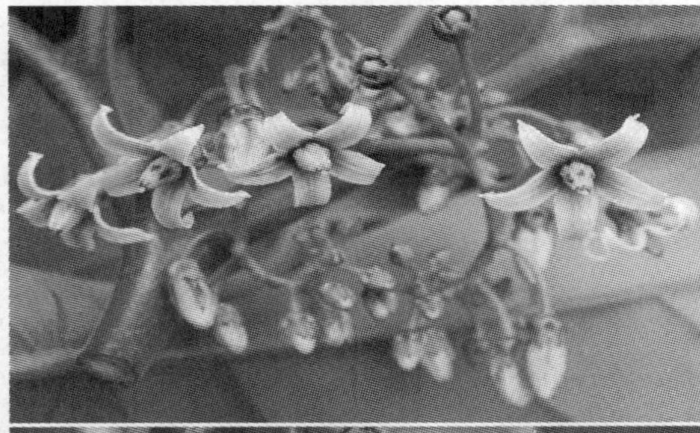

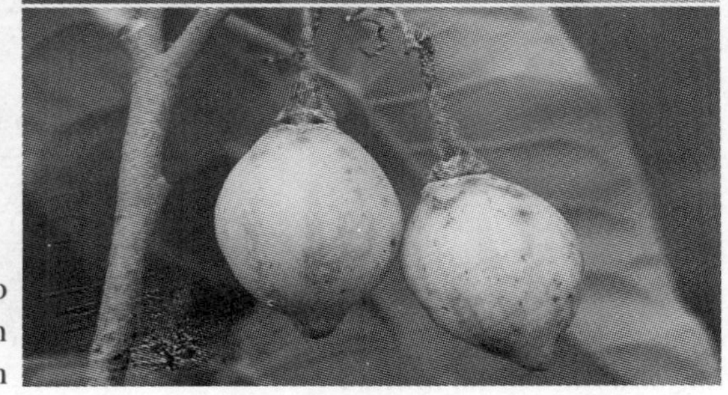

Family:
Solanaceae **(Potato family)**

Common Names:
Indian nightshade • Hindi: *Barhati, Barhatta* • Manipuri: *Leipungkhangga* • Tamil: *Karimulli* • Malayalam: *Puttiriccunta*

Description:
A much branched shrub 0.3-1.5 m high, with large prickles. Stem stout,often purple. Branches covered with minute stellate hairs. Leaves 5-15 by 2.5-7.5 cm ovate in outline,acute,clothed with simple hairs. Flowers in racemose extra axillary cymes, purple coloured, clothed with darker purple coloured hairs. Fruit berry 8 mm diameter globose, dark yellow, when ripe. Seeds minutely pitted.

Medicinal Uses:
In Manipur, ***a paste of the Indian nightshade fruit with honey*** is administered as a medicine for ***high fever.***

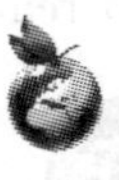

Black Nightshade

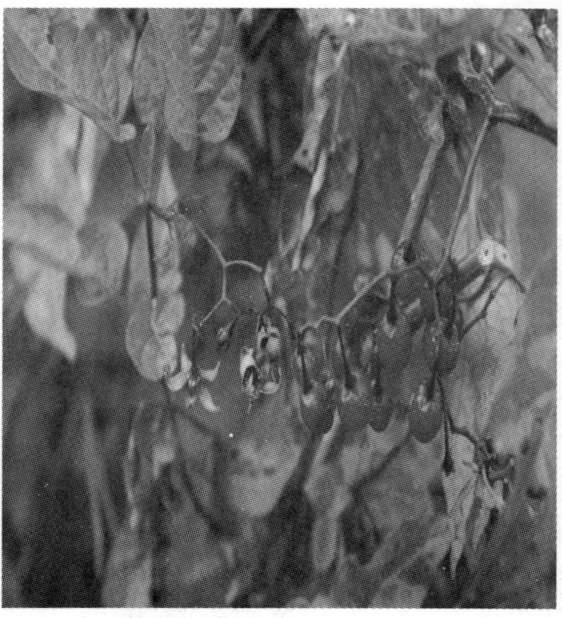

Botanical Name:
Solanum nigrum

Family:
Solanaceae **(Potato family)**

Common Names:
Black nightshade, Black-berry night shade, Nightshade, Poisonberry • Manipuri: *Leipungkhangga* • Tamil: *Manatakkali* • Hindi: *Mokoi* • Malayalam: *Mulakuthakkali* • Telugu: *Kasaka* • Marathi: *Laghukavali* • Urdu: *Makoya*

Description:
Black Nightshade is a plant, an annual weed that grows up to 60cm tall, is branched and usually erect, growing wild in wastelands and crop fields. Alternate leaves are ovate deep green with an indented margin and acuminate at the tip. Flowers are white with yellow coloured center. The berries are green at early stage and turn to orange or black when ripened.

Medicinal Uses:
Black Nightshade is used for *skin diseases, rheumatism* and *gouts.* The *juice of the herb* is given in *chronic enlargement of the liver.* It can *cure ear and eye diseases.* It is sometimes prescribed to 'remove the effects of old age'.

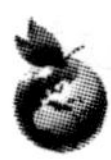

Thorny Nightshade

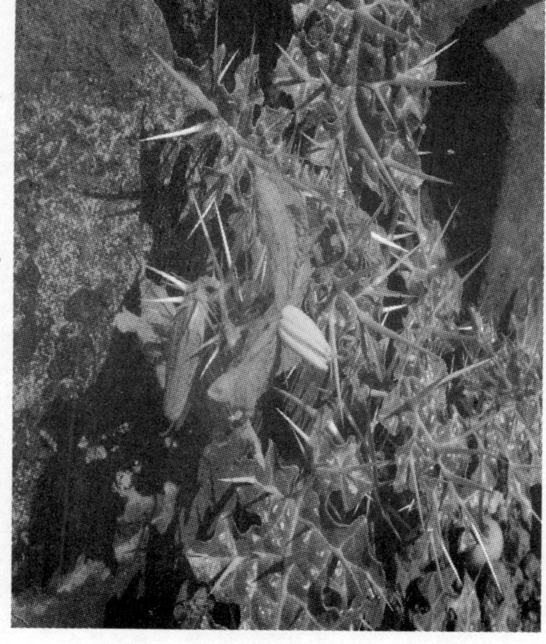

Botanical Name:
Solanum virginianum

Family:
Solanaceae **(Potato family)**

Synonyms:
Solanum surattense, Solanum xanthocarpum

Common Names:
Thorny Nightshade, Yellow Berried Nightshade, Thai eggplant • Hindi: *Kateli, Oonth Kateli* • Manipuri: *Leipungkhanga* • Marathi: *Kateringani* • Tamil: *Kantankattiri* • Malayalam: *Kantakariccunta, Kantakarivalutana* • Telugu: *Nelamulaka, Vakudu* • Kannada: *Kantikari* • Bengali: *Kantakari* • Oriya: *Bheji-baigana* • Konkani: *Kante ringini* • Sanskrit: *Kantakari*

Description:
Thorny Nightshade is a herb which is erect or creeping, sometimes woody at base, 50-70 cm tall, copiously armed with sturdy, needlelike, broad-based prickles 0.5-2 cm × 0.5-1.5 mm.

Leaves are unequal paired; stalk 2-3.5 cm, prickly; leaf blade ovate-oblong, 4-9 × 2-4.5 cm, prickly along veins, margin usually 5-9-lobed or pinnately parted, lobes unequal, sinuate, apex acute.

Inflorescences elongate racemes 4-7 cm. Sepal tube is bell-shaped 1 cm in diameter.

Flowers blue-purple, 1.4-1.6 × 2.5 cm; petals ovate-deltate, 6-8 mm, densely pubescent with stellate hairs.

Filaments 1 mm; anthers 8 mm. Style 1 cm. Fruiting pedicel 2-3.6 cm, with prickles and sparse stellate hairs.

Fruiting sepals prickly, sparsely pubescent. Berry pale yellow, 1.3-2.2 cm in diameter. Flowering: November-May.

Medicinal Uses:

Boiled decoction of the dry plant is prescribed for *stomach and liver complaints.*

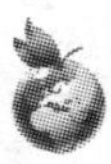

Ashwagandha

Botanical Name:
Withania somnifera

Family:
Solanaceae **(Potato family)**

Common Names:
Winter Cherry • Hindi: *Ashwagandha, Rasbhari* • Kannada: *Kanchuki* • Marathi: *Ghoda, Tilli* • Gujarati: *Ghodaasun* • Telugu: *Vajigandha* • Malayalam: *Amukkuram* • Tamil: *Amukkuram*

Description:
Ashwagandha, is native to drier parts of India. It is a perennial herb that reaches about 6 feet in nature. In the greenhouse they flower in the late fall and winter. Orange fruits in persistent papery calyxes follow the small greenish flowers. Ashwagandha is propagated by division, cuttings or seed. Seed is the best way to propagate them. Seed sown on moist sand will germinate in 14-21 days at 20° C.

Medicinal Uses:
Ashwagandha has been a prized as a top-notch *adaptogenic tonic in India for 3000 - 4000 years.* The plants contain the *alkaloids* withanine and somniferine, which are used to treat *nervous disorders, intestinal infections* and *leprosy.* All *plant parts* are used including the *roots, bark, leaves, fruits* and *seeds.*

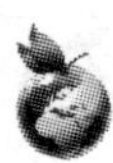

Apple Mangrove

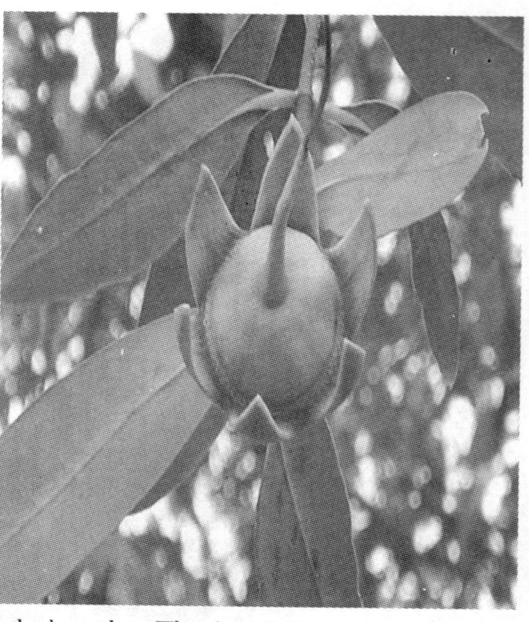

Botanical Name:

Sonneratia caseolaris

Family:

Sonneratiaceae **(Apple mangrove family)**

Common Names:

Apple Mangrove, Crabapple mangrove

Description:

Apple mangrove is a small evergreen tree, upto 8.0 m high, numerous branches, woody, erect, branches horizontal, twig slender. Leaves are about 7 cm long, rounded and opposite each other on the branches. The tips of the leaves are slightly turned under. Sonneratia alba has white flowers while Sonneratia caseolaris has red flowers. Sepal tube is green with 6 valvular lobes. There are 6 red petals, which are overshadowed by long showy, numerous stamens, which are white, but reddish at the base. Flowers only open for one night and have an offensive smell. The fruit are large (4 cm wide) green, leathery berries with a star-shaped base. When ripe, the fruits are eaten raw or cooked.

Medicinal Uses:

Fermented fruit juice is said to be useful in *arresting haemorrhage.* The wall of an old fruit is given as a *vermifuge.* The juice of half-ripe fruit is used to *treat coughs.* The juice of the flowers enters into a compound for *treating blood in the urine.*

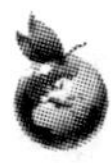

Devil`s Cotton

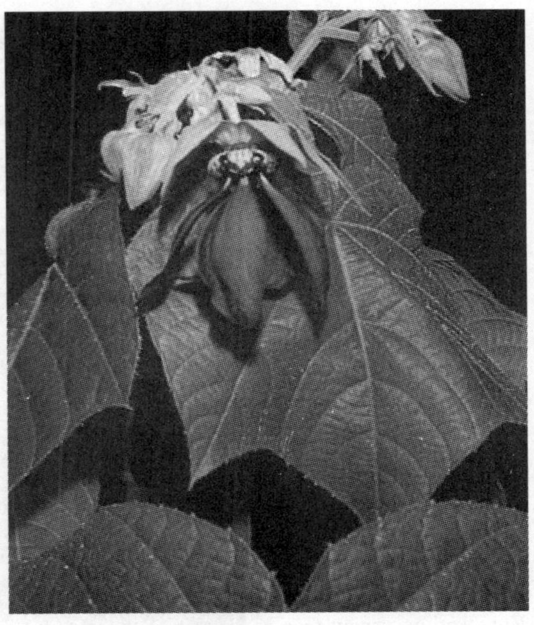

Botanical Name:
Abroma angusta

Family:
Sterculiaceae **(Cacao family)**

Common Names:
Devil's Cotton, Cotton Abroma • Nepali: *Chinne, Sanu kapase, Ulatkambal, Pisach karpas*

Description:
Devil's Cotton is a large spreading shrub, or a small tree, with fibrous bark and irritant hairs. It grows up to 2.5 m tall with hairy branches. Leaves are ovate-oblong long-pointed, with a heart-shaped base, 10-21 cm long, 5.5-13 cm wide. Leaf blade is 3-7 nerved, with margins unevenly toothed. Flowers are maroon, up to 5 cm across, looking down, in few-flowered clusters in leaf axils. Sepals are lance- shaped, fused at base. Petals are 5, which soon fall off, concave below, prolonged above into a spoon-shaped blade. Capsule is papery, 5-winged, cut-off at the tip. The fibre from the bark makes a pliable and attractive rope which is used in fishing nets. Devil's Cotton is found in the Himalayas and NE India. Flowering: June-September.

Medicinal Uses:
The *fresh viscid sap of the root bark* is considered to be a valuable *emenagogue* and *uterine tonic.* The *root* has also been applied to *treat skin rashes* and *itches.*

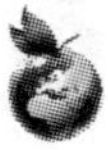

East-Indian Screw Tree

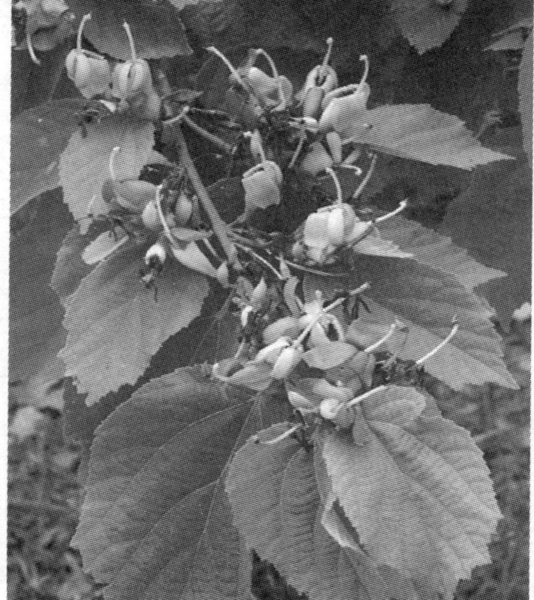

Botanical Name:
Helicteres isora

Family:
Sterculiaceae **(Cacao family)**

Common Names:
East-Indian screw tree, Nut-leaved screw tree

- Hindi: *Maror phali*
- Marathi: *Murud sheng*
- Sanskrit: *Mriga Shringa*
- Kannada: *Yedmuri*
- Telugu: *Valambiri*
- Tamil: *Vadampiri*
- Bengali: *Antamora*

Description:
East-Indian screw tree is a sub-deciduous shrub or small tree with grey coloured bark. Leaves simple, serrate margin, scabrous above and pubescent beneath. Flowers solitary or in sparse clusters, with red petals turning pale blue when old. Fruits greenish brown, beaked, cylindrical, spirally twisted on ripening. The twisted shape of the fruit is what lends most of its names like screw tree and *maror phali.*

Medicinal Uses:
The *roots and stem barks* are considered to be *expectorant, demulcent, astringent* and *antiglactagogue.* The bark is used in *diarrhoea, dysentery, biliousness* and is useful in *gripping of the bowels.* Root juice is used in *antidiarrhoeal* and *antidysenteric formulations. Fried pods* are given to *children* to *kill intestinal worms.*

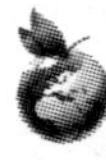

Guest Tree

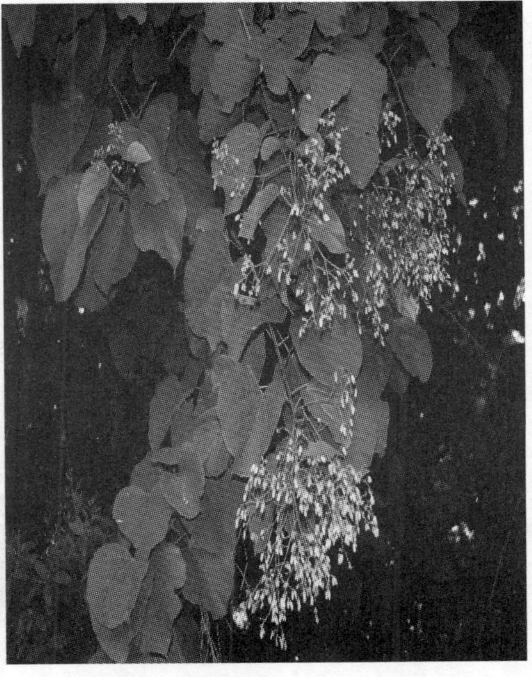

Botanical Name:
Kleinhovia hospita

Family:
Sterculiaceae **(Cacao family)**

Common Names:
Guest Tree, Timanga tree • Hindi: *Bhola* • Bengali: *Bola*

Description:
Guest Tree is an evergreen, bushy tree growing up to 20 m high, with a dense rounded crown and upright pink sprays of flowers and fruits. It grows from 8 to 15 m in height. The leaves are broadly ovate, and 10-20 cm long, with pointed tip, and heart-shaped base. The flowers are pink, about 8 mm long, and borne in panicles 20-40 cm long, terminating the branches. The fruit is a thin-walled, inflated capsule about 2 cm long. The young leaves are eaten as a green. The bast fiber is widely used for tying bundles. It is also made into rope which is used for tethering carabaos and horses, and for making halters. The rope is said to be durable during rainy weather.

Medicinal Uses:
Guest Tree is used as a *traditional medicine* in parts of *Malaya, Indonesia* and *Papua New Guinea* to treat *scabies.* The *bark* and *leaves are* used as *hairwash* for *lice*, while the *juice of the leaves* are used as an *eyewash.*

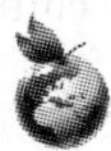

Fiji Arrowroot

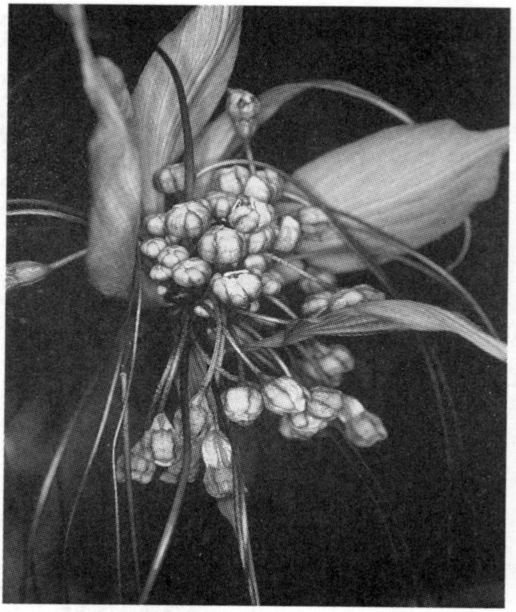

Botanical Name:
Tacca leontopetaloides

Family:
Taccaceae **(Bat Flower family)**

Synonyms:
Tacca hawaiiensis, Tacca involucrata, Tacca pinnatifida

Common Names:
Fiji Arrowroot, Batflower, East Indian arrowroot, Polynesian arrowroot, Tahiti arrowroot • Hindi: *Bagh-moochh, Devkanda* • Marathi: *Devkanda* • Tamil: *Cenai, Kakanam, Kattu-k-karunai* • Telugu: *Adavidumpa*

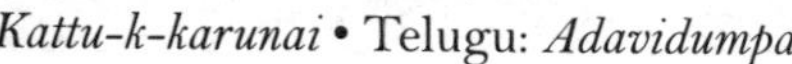

Description:
Fiji Arrowroot is a perennial herb naturally distributed from western Africa through southeast Asia to northern Australia. The leaf's upper surface has depressed veins, and the under surface is shiny with bold yellow veins.

Greenish purple flowers are borne on tall stalks in clusters, with long trailing whisker-like bracts. The plant is usually dormant for part of the year and dies down to the ground.

Later, new leaves will arise from the round underground tuber. The tubers are hard and potato-like, with a brown skin and white interior.

The tubers of Polynesian arrowroot contain starch that was an important food source for many Pacific Island cultures, primarily for the inhabitants of low islands and atolls. Polynesian arrowroot was prepared into a flour to make a variety of puddings.

Medicinal Uses:

In *traditional Hawaiian medicine*, the *raw tubers* were eaten to treat *stomach ailments*. Mixed with water and red clay, the plant was consumed to treat *diarrhoea* and *dysentery*.

This combination was also used to stop *internal haemorrhaging* in the *stomach* and *colon* and *applied to wounds* to *stop bleeding*.

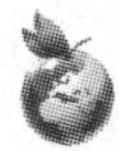

Elegant False Tamarisk

Botanical Name:
Tamaricaria elegans

Family:
Tamaricaceae **(Tamarisk family)**

Synonyms:
Myricaria elegans, Myrtama elegans

Common Names:
Elegant False Tamarisk, Myricaria, False tamarisk

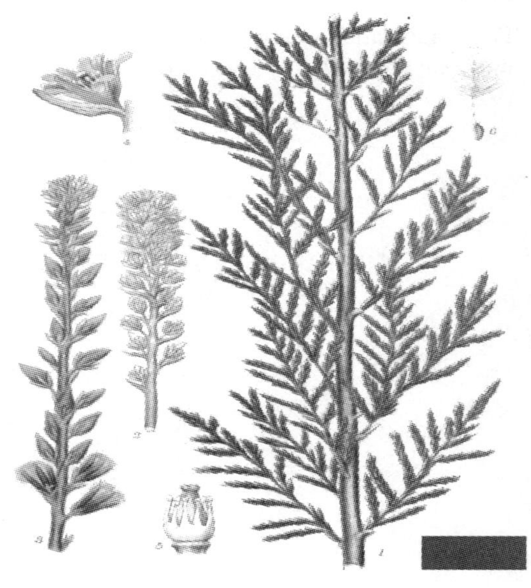

Description:
Elegant False Tamarisk is a deciduous erect shrub that grows to 5 m tall. Old branches red-brown or dark purple, branches of current year green or red-brown. Leaves usually in green branchlets of current year, sessile, narrowly elliptic, elliptic-lanceolate, or ovate-lanceolate, relatively large, 5-15 × 2-3 mm, base narrow, margin narrowly membranous, apex obtuse or acute. Flower racemes usually lateral, rarely at the end of branches. Petals white, pink or purple-red, obovate, obovate-elliptic, or elliptic, or narrowly obovate or obovate-lanceolate, to 5-6 × 2-3 mm, base gradually narrowing, apex obtuse. Stamens slightly shorter than petals. It grows gregariously by streams, riversides, sandy places at lakesides, at altitudes of 3000-4300 m. Flowering: June-July.

Medicinal Uses:
The *leaves* are used *externally* as a *poultice on bruises.*

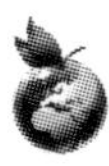

Phalsa

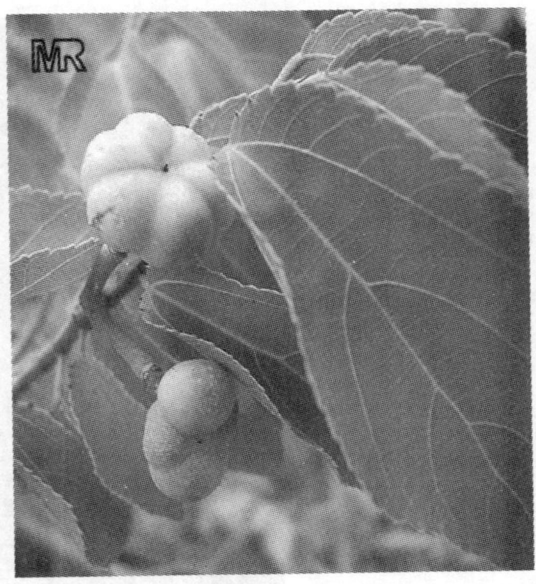

Botanical Name:

Grewia asiatica

Family:

Tiliaceae **(Phalsa family)**

Common Names:

Hindi, Urdu, Marathi: *Phalsa* • Kannada: *Phulsha* • Telugu: *Phutiki* • Sindhi: *Pharaho* • Konkani: *Phalsi* • Gujarati: *Shukri* • Sanskrit: *Mriduphal* • Oriya: *Pharosakoli* • Malayalam: *Chadicha* • Tamil: *Unnu*

Description:

Phalsa is a shrub or small tree which can grow upto 12 feet high. Its bark is greyish-white or greyish-brown. Leaves with serrated margins vary from broadly heart-shaped to obliquely ovate. The flowers are yellow about 2 centimetres in length, and borne in densely crowded (rarely solitary) axillary cymes. The fruit is edible, rounded, small dark blue to almost black when ripe, sweetish and somewhat acidic, with a fairly good flavour and each fruit contains a rather large seed. The fruit is eaten raw with relish and sold in Delhi lanes in summers, with great enthusiasm by singing hawkers.

Medicinal Uses:

The *fruit* is supposed to possess *astringent, cooling* and *stomachic properties. A spirit is distilled* and a *pleasant sherbet* is made from it. The leaves are used as an application to *pustular eruptions.* The Indian Santals a jungle tribe prescribe the *root-bark* for *rheumatism.* In Sind, *an infusion of the bark* is used as a *demulcent.*

Indian Elm

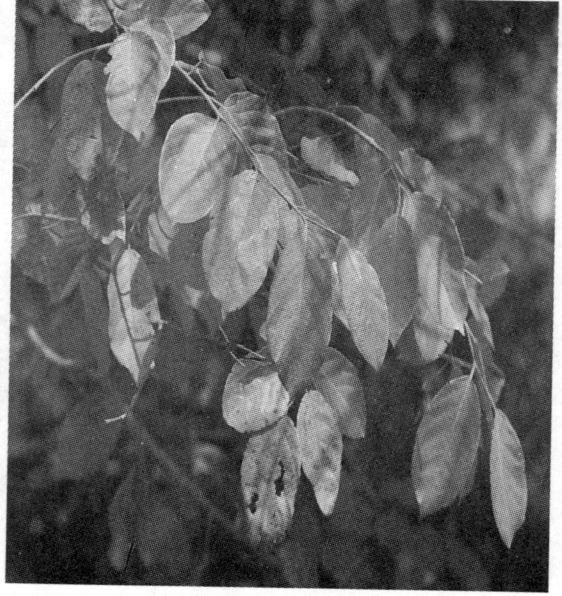

Botanical Name:
Holoptelea integrifolia

Family:
Ulmaceae **(Elm family)**

Synonyms:
Ulmus integrifolia

Common Names:
Indian Elm, Entire-leaved elm tree, Jungle cork tree, South Indian elm tree • Hindi: *Chilbil, Kanju, Papri* • Marathi: *Ainasadada, or Vavala* • Tamil: *Aya* • Malayalam: *Aaval* • Telugu: *Nali* • Bengali *Nata karanja* • Oriya: *Dhauranjan* • Konkani: *Vamvlo* • Gujarati: *Charal, Charel, Kanjo* • Sanskrit: *Chirivilva* • Nepali: *Sano pangro*

Description:
Indian Elm is a large deciduous tree, growing up to 18 m tall. It has grey bark, covered with blisters, peeling in corky scales on old trees.

Alternately arranged leaves are elliptic-ovate, 8-13 cm long and 3.2-6.3 cm wide, smooth, with entire margins and a pointed tip.

Leaf base is rounded or heart-shaped. Stipules are lance-shaped. Crushed leaves emit an unpleasant odour.

Flowers are small, greenish-yellow to brownish, pubescent, borne in short racemes or fascicles at the scars of fallen leaves.

Sepals are velvety, often four. The fruit is an a circular samara, 2.5 cm in diameter, with membranous, net-veined wings, and flat seeds.

Medicinal Uses:

The *bark of the Indian Elm* is used in *rheumatism.* Seeds and *paste of the stem and bark* is used in *treating ringworms.*

Bark and leaves are used for treating *oedema, diabetes, leprosy* and other *skin diseases, intestinal disorders* and *piles.*

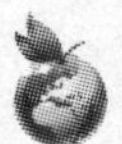

Bichchhoo

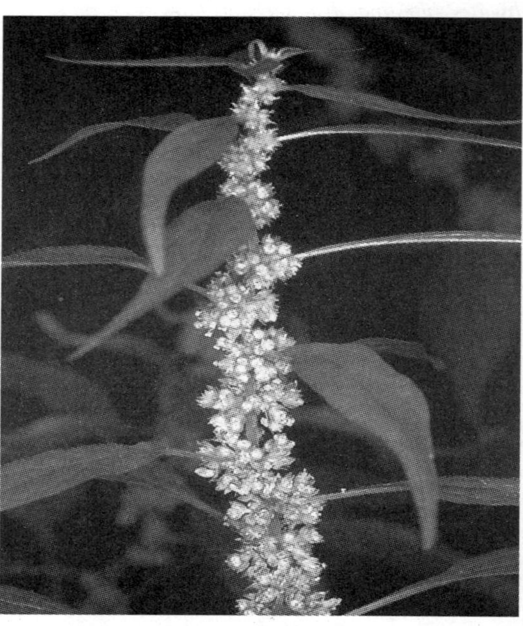

Botanical Name:
Girardiana platyphylla

Family:
Urticaceae **(Nettle family)**

Synonyms:
Urtica heterophylla

Common Names:
Bichchhoo, Indian Stinging nettle • Hindi: *Bichchhoo* • Manipuri: *Santhak*

Description:
This is a much despised plant in the hills of North India due to is very virulent stinging hairs. The plant grows to heights of 3 or 4 feet and is often used as fencing to keep out cattle. The popular Hindi name *Bichchhoo* which is means *scorpion.* Indeed the itch produced by the plant, which in milder doses is that of many red ants, and with extensive contact can be like that of bees or scorpion stings, and may need anti-allergic medication. The itch is produced from the formic acid contained in the oil glands under the stinging hairs.

Medicinal Uses:
However, the plant itself has medicinal value and *Nettle Tea* has been used in Europe for many centuries. The *leaves should not be touched with bare hands, but dried or boiled thoroughly in water*, and are used as *diuretic, anti- rheumatic, anti-allergic* and also for *lactating mothers.* The other parts of the plant are also useful for the production of *oils, biomass* and *fibres or paper.*

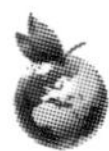

Indian Valerian

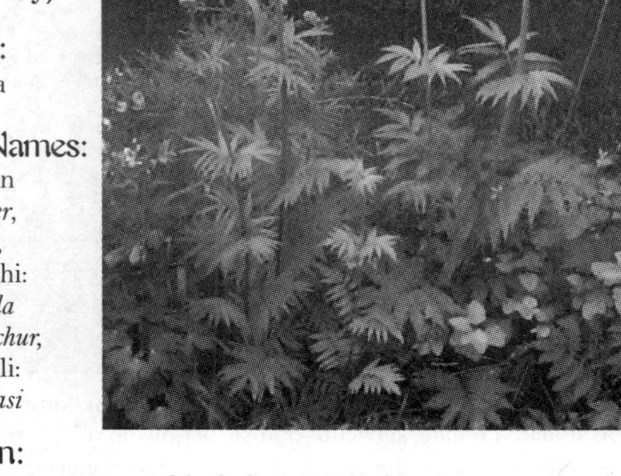

Botanical Name:
Valeriana hardwickii

Family:
Valerianaceae
(Valeriana family)

Synonyms:
Valeriana elata

Common Names:
Indian Valerian
• Hindi: *Tagger, Asarun, Shami, Chhar* • Marathi: *Taggerganthoda* • Bengali: *Balchur, Tagger* • Nepali: *Nakkali jatamasi*

Description:
Indian Valerian is a *perennial herb*, distinguished by its 1-3 pairs of stem-leaves which are large, compound, with 3-5 leaflets, and its white or pale pink flowers. These tiny flower, 2-3 mm across, are borne in dense, domed clusters at the end of branches. The clusters form a branched pyramidal inflorescence. Basal leaves are long-stalked, and are usually shriveled during flowering. Stem is 1-6 ft tall. Indian Valerian is found in shrubberies and open slopes, at altitudes of 1500-4000 m. Flowering: June-September.

Medicinal Uses:
Indian Valerian is a well-known and frequently used *medicinal herb* that has a long and proven history of efficacy. It is noted especially for its effect as a *tranquilliser* and *nervine*, particularly for those people suffering from *nervous overstrain.* Valerian has been shown to *encourage sleep, improve sleep quality* and *reduce blood pressure.*

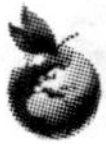

Arni

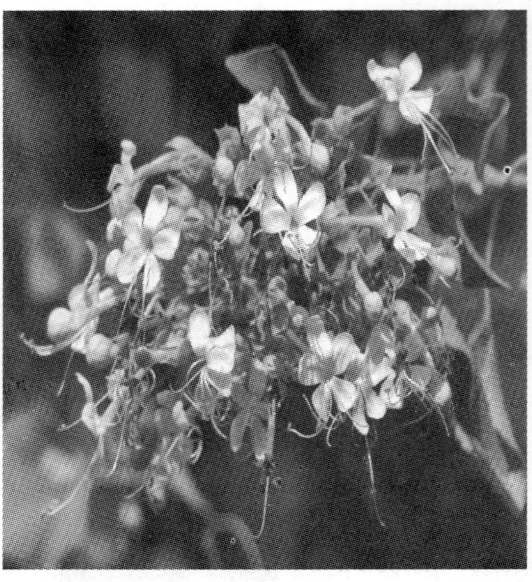

Botanical Name:
Clerodendrum phlomidis

Family:
Verbenaceae **(Verbena family)**

Common Names:
Hindi: *Arni* • Kannada: *Taggi gida* • Tamil: *Taluddai*

Description:
A fairly common shrub of arid plains, low hills, deserts of Sind, Punjab and Baluchistan. Shrubs 1.5-3 m tall, stem ashy-grey, branches pubescent. Leaves opposite, ovate to rhomboid-ovate, 1.5-5 cm long, 1-3 cm broad, entire to sinuate-crenate, subacute-obtuse; petiole up to 2.5 cm long. Flowers creamy-white or pale yellowish, c. 1.5 cm across; pedicels 5-10 mm long, densely hirsute; bracts ovate lanceolate. Calyx campanulate, glabrous, pale or somewhat yellowish green, somewhat inflated, 5-lobed; lobes 4-5 mm long, ovate-triangulate, Corolla-tube 2-2.5 cm long, much narrower than the calyx, pubescent externally; lobes 5, subequal, ovate-elliptic, 7-8 mm long, obtuse. Drupe obovoid, 8-12 mm long, black, wrinkled, usually 4-lobed, enclosed by the persistent calyx; seeds oblong, white. Distribution: Pakistan, India, Sri Lanka and Burma.

Medicinal Uses:
The *root* is used as a *bitter tonic* and given in *convalescence of measles.* The *juice of leaves* is alterative and given in *neglected syphilitic complaints.* The *root* is given as a *demulcent* in *gonorrhoea,* and the *decoction of the plant* is considered as an *alternative.* It helps to cure *stomach problems* and *swellings in cattle.*

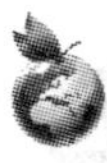

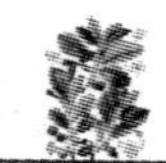

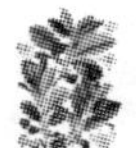

Hill Glory Bower

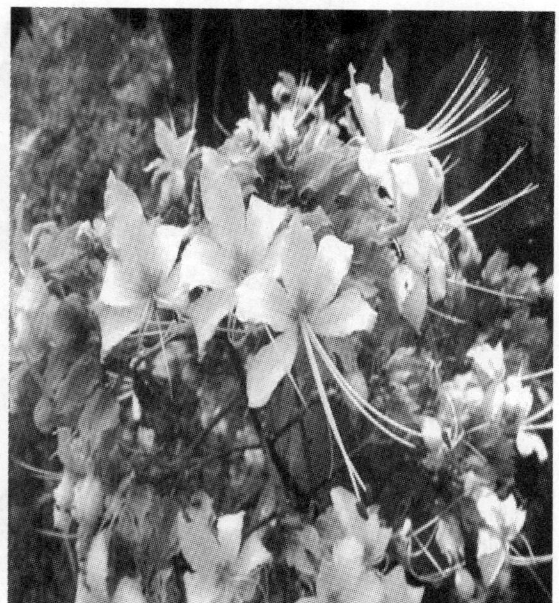

Botanical Name:
Clerodendrum viscosum

Family:
Verbenaceae **(Verbena family)**

Common Names:
Hill Glory Bower • Hindi: *Titabhamt, Bhant* • Manipuri: *Kuthap manbi* • Marathi: *Bhandira* • Tamil: *Perukilai* • Malayalam: *Peruku* • Telugu: *Gurrapu katilyaku* • Kannada: *Ibbane, Basavana pada* • Bengali: *Bhant* • Sanskrit: *Bhandirah* • Nepali: *Rajbeli*

Description:
Hill glory bower is a *gregarious shrub, 1-2 m high.* The quadrangular branches are covered with sily yellwish hair. Oppositely arranged leaves are oval, 10-20 cm long, hairy. The base of the leaf is heart-shaped. White flowers, tinged with pink, occur in large panicles. The five white petals are tinged pink at the base. Four long stamens, 3 cm, protrude out of the flower. Flowering: March-April.

Medicinal Uses:
The *extract of the leaves* is given *orally in fever* and *bowel troubles* in the Kuki and Rongmei tribes in the *North-East India.* The fresh *leaf-juice* is introduced in the *rectum for the removal of ascarids.* The *leaves and flowers* are used to cure *scorpion sting.*

Gamhar

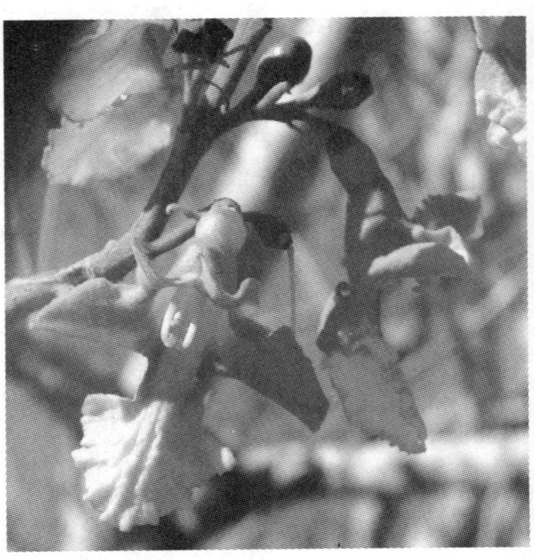

Botanical Name:

Gmelina arborea

Family:

Verbenaceae **(Verbena family)**

Common Names:

Gamhar • Hindi: *Gamhar* • Manipuri: *Wang* • Marathi: *Sivan* • Tamil: *Kumalaamaram* • Malayalam: *Kumbil* • Telugu: *Peddagumudutekku* • Kannada: *Shivani* • Konkani: *Sirni* • Sanskrit: *Madhumati*

Description:

Gamhar is a *beautiful fast growing deciduous tree* occurring naturally throughout greater part of India up to 1500 m. It is a fast growing tree, which though grows on different localities and prefers moist fertile valleys with 7500-4500 mm rainfall.

It does not thrive on ill drained soils and remains stunted on dry, sandy or poor soils; drought also reduces it to a shrubby form. The tree attains moderate to large height up to 30 m with girth of 1.2 to 4.5 m with a clear bole of 9-15 m. It is a treat to see the gamhar tree standing straight with clear bole having branches on top and thick foliage forming a conical crown on the top of the tall stem.

Bark light grey coloured exfoliating in light coloured patches when old, blaze thick, a chlorophyll layer just under the outer bark, pale yellow white inside.

Flowering takes place during February to April when the tree is more or less leafless whereas fruiting starts from May onwards up to June. Flowers occur in narrow branching clusters at the end of branches. The yellow flower, tinged with brown, is trumpet shaped, 3-4 cm long. The trumpets flare open into a gaping mouth with distinct lobes.

Medicinal Uses:

The *root and bark* of Gmelina *arborea* are *stomachic, galactagogue laxative* and *anthelmintic,* improves *appetite,* useful in removing *hallucination, piles, abdominal pains, burning sensations, fevers, 'tridosha'* and *urinary discharge.* The leaf paste is applied to relieve headache and juice is used as a wash for ulcers. *Flowers* are *sweet, cooling, bitter, acrid and astringent.*

They are useful in *leprosy* and *blood diseases.* In *Ayurveda,* it has been observed that the Gamhar fruit is *acrid, sour, bitter, sweet, cooling, diuretic tonic, aphrodisiac, alternative astringent to the bowels,* promote growth of *hairs, useful in 'vata', thirst, anaemia, leprosy, ulcers* and *vaginal discharge.*

The plant is recommended in combination with other drugs for the treatment of *snake – bites* and *scorpion- stings.* In snake–bites, a *decoction of the roots* and *bark* is given *internally.*

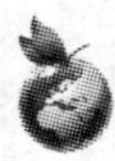

Frog Fruit

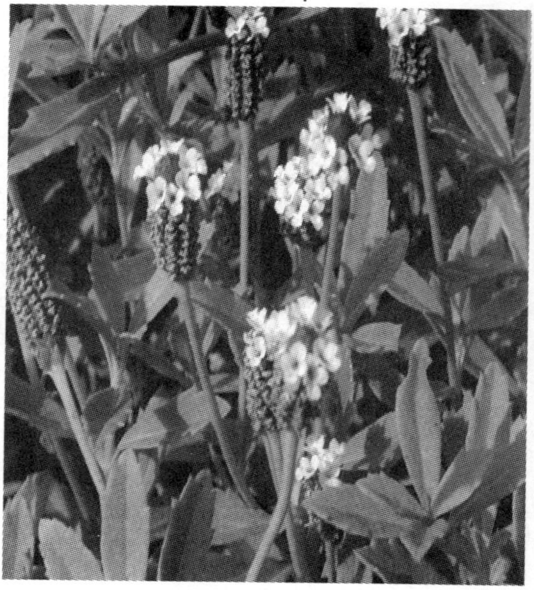

Botanical Name:
Phyla nodiflora

Family:
Verbenaceae **(Verbena family)**

Common Names:
Frog Fruit, Turkey Tangle, Creeping Lip Plant, Lippia
- Hindi: *Jal buti, Jalpapli*
- Manipuri: *Chinglengbi*
- Marathi: *Jalapimpali*
- Tamil: *Podutalei*
- Malayalam: *Nirtippali*
- Telugu: *Bokkena*
- Kannada: *Nelahippali*
- Konkani: *Adali*

Description:
Frog Fruit is a flowering, broadleaf plant native to South America. It is grows in a groundcover or turflike manner, and is often present in yards. The inflorescence consists of a purple-coloured center encircled by small white-to-pink flowers. The flower takes on a match-like look, which is why the plant is called matchweed. The leaf arrangement is opposite. Each leaf has one to seven teeth on each edge starting at the widest point and continuing to the tip.

Medicinal Uses:
The *Plant decoction* is given in *uraema. Fresh juice* is applied to *bleeding gums.* The *Infusion of leaves and tender stalk* is given to *children* in *indigestion* and to *women after delivery.*

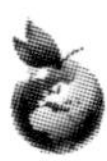

Vervain

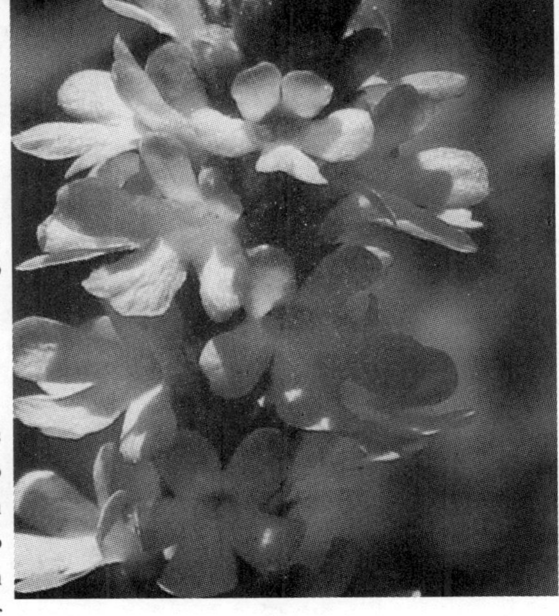

Botanical Name:

Verbena officinalis

Family:

Verbenaceae **(Verbena family)**

Common Names:

Vervain, Simpler's Joy, European vervain, Herb of Grace • Manipuri: *Tharo-phijub*

Description:

Vervain is a herbaceous perennial thought to originate in Southern Europe through to China but has been widely grown for thousands of years by many cultures.

Has mid-green, slightly hairy, lobed, almost diamond shaped leaves. Bears tiny, lilac, 2 lipped flowers with a larger, 5 lobed bottom lip, borne on slender flower spikes.

The flowers open from the bottom of the spike first. It rarely has more then 4 flowers open on the spike at any one time so it's quite inconspicuous unless you look for it.

Flowers June-October but may open as early as April. Once considered a very sacred herb. The druids supposedly introduced it to the Romans.

The Romans so venerated the plant they even held an annual festival in honour of it called Verbenalia.

Roman brides also wore the flowers at weddings as it was sacred to the goddess of love Venus.

Medicinal Uses:

Vervain makes an excellent *nerve tonic* and is used in the treatment of *nervous disorders, epilepsy, some respiratory problems,* such as *whooping cough, urinary tract problems, sedative, detoxification, as a digestive,* a *cooling wash for mild fever, sore throats, some skin complaints* like *eczema* and for bringing out bruising.

It can also be used as a *refreshing eye tonic* and surprisingly, it was one of the *first commercial hair tonics.*

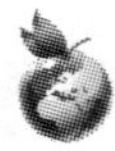

Chaste Tree

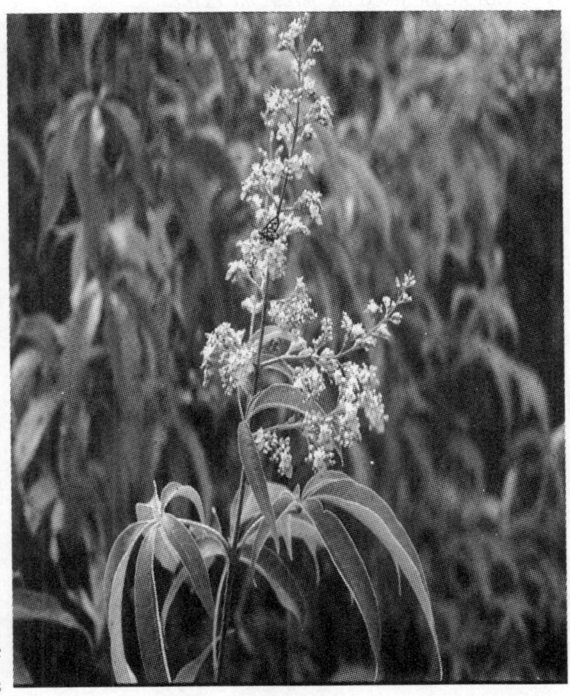

Botanical Name:

Vitex negundo

Family:

Verbenaceae **(Verbena family)**

Common Names:

Chaste Tree • Hindi: *Nirgundi, Sindvar* • Manipuri: *Urik shibi* • Tamil: *Nocchi* • Malayalam: *Vennocchi* • Telugu: *Vavili* • Kannada: *Nochi* • Bengali: *Samalu*

Description:

Chaste tree can be described as a cross between a shrub and a tree with a single woody stem (trunk). It can grow up to five metres tall.

Chaste tree's distinctive feature are the pointed leaves with 3-5 leaflets. Small, lilac or violet flowers on new growth from June to September. Flowers are the smallest of the commonly grown Vitex species.

The leaves are used as a *mosquito repellent.* leaves are burnt in a heap which proves very useful to get rid of mosquitoes.

Medicinal Uses:

It is an effective *herbal medicine* with proven *therapeutic value.*

Chaste Tree has been clinically tested to be effective in the treatment of *colds, flu, asthma* and *pharyngitis.* Studies have shown that it can prevent the body's production of *leukotrienes,* which are released during an *asthma attack.*

The Chaste Tree contains *Chrysoplenol D*, a substance with *anti-histamine properties* and *muscle relaxant.* The *leaves, flowers, seeds* and *roots* of a Chaste tree can all be used as *herbal medicine.*

A *decoction* is made by *boiling the parts of the plant* and taken orally. Today, a Chaste Tree is available in *capsule form* and *syrup for cough.*

Spade Flower

Botanical Name:
Hybanthus enneaspermus

Family:
Violaceae **(Violet family)**

Synonyms:
Ionidium suffruticosum

Common Names:
Spade Flower, Pink ladies slipper • Hindi: *Ratan purush* • Bengali: *Munbora* • Kannada: *Purusharathna* •Malayalam: *Orilathamatai* • Telugu: *Ratnapurusha* • Marathi: *Rathanparas* • Sanskrit: *Rathnapurusha*

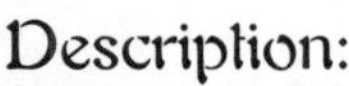

Description:
Spade Flower is a perennial herb or small shrub to 60 cm high, smooth or hairy. Leaves are linear to lance-like, 1-5 cm long, margins recurved to revolute, occasionally flat; stipules acuminate, 1-4 mm long. Pink-purple spade-shaped flowers occur solitary.

Sepals 3-4 mm long. Lower petal broad spade-shaped, pink-purple, with deep purple veins. Upper petals linear-oblong, 3-4 mm long; lateral pair 4.5-5 mm long.

Anthers without appendages. Capsule 4-9 mm long; seeds 5-12, pitted between ribs.

Medicinal Uses:

This *herb* is considered to be extremely beneficial to men, used as *a diuretic, demulcent* and *tonic.*

The *root* is *diuretic* and is used in *urinary affections* and *bowel complaints* of children. *Decoction* of *leaves* and *tender stalks* is *demulcent.*

The fruit is used to treat *scorpion sting.* It is a *hard task to collect adequate quantities of whole plants,* let *alone individual parts.*

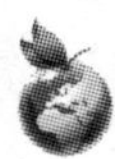

Leafless Mistletoe

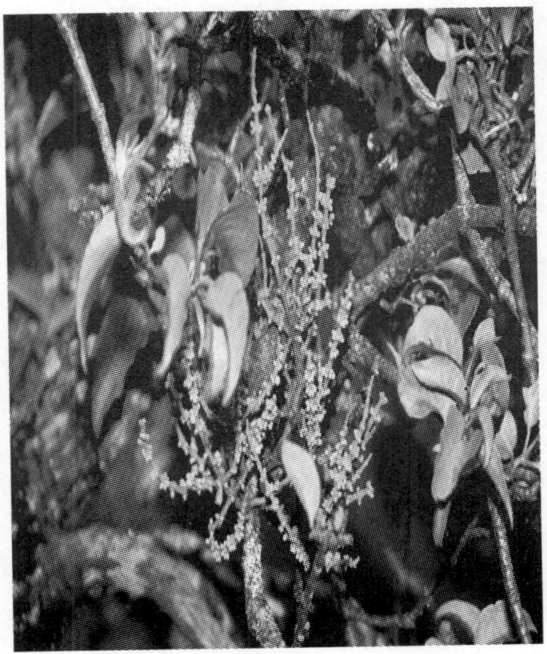

Botanical Name:

Viscum articulatum

Family:

Viscaceae **(Mistletoe family)**

Synonyms:

Viscum nepalense

Common Names:

Leafless Mistletoe, Jointed Mistletoe • Hindi: *Budu, Pudu, Hurchu* • Mizo: *Lenpat* • Marathi: *Banda* • Kannada: *Badanike* • Bengali: *Mandala* • Oriya: *Madanga* • Gujarati: *Vando* • Sanskrit: *Kamini*

Description:

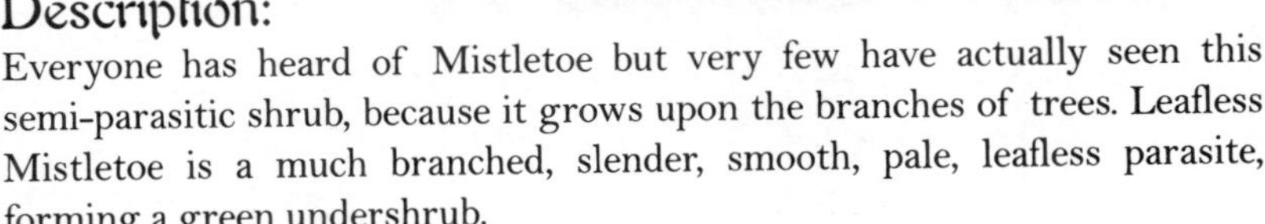

Everyone has heard of Mistletoe but very few have actually seen this semi-parasitic shrub, because it grows upon the branches of trees. Leafless Mistletoe is a much branched, slender, smooth, pale, leafless parasite, forming a green undershrub.

The branches are flat, with pendulous tufts, 15-90 cm long; the internodes being variable in length; usually a trifle wider at the distal end, and striate. The leaves are visible only in the very young internodes as small bracts below the flowers.

The flowers are very minute, stalkless, and in stalkless, 3-flowered spikes. There are two or several spikes at a joint.

The perianth of the male flowers is reflexed, and hardly ¼ mm long. The female flowers are about 1/2 mm long, with two bracts, and the perianth lobes erect and triangular.

The fruit is stalkless, nearly spherical, about 3 mm in diameter, white and shining when ripe. In Europe the mistletoe is well known for the Christmas custom of kissing beneath its branches.

It also features in the popular Asterix comic books, where mistletoe collected from oaks was considered to have special qualities. Flowering: December-January.

Medicinal Uses:

Leafless Mistletoe is used as a *cure for fever. The paste* is applied to *cuts.*

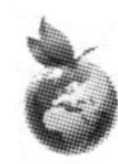

Bush Grape

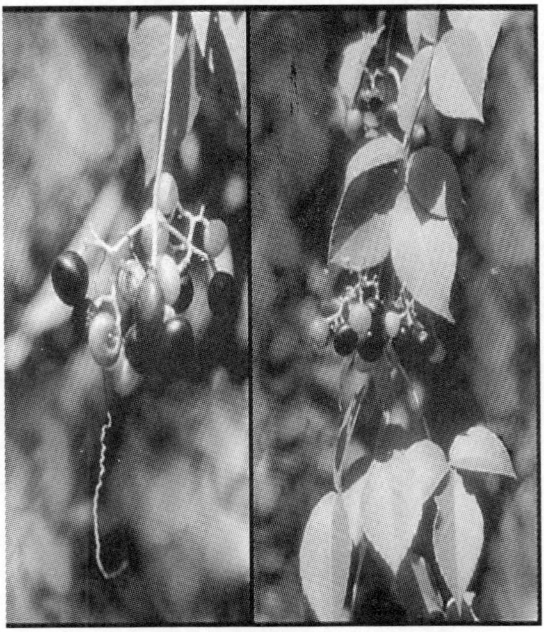

Botanical Name:
Cayratia trifolia

Family:
Vitaceae **(Grape family)**

Synonyms:
Cissus trifolia, Vitis trifolia, Vitis carnosa

Common Names:
Bush Grape, Fox-grape, Three-leaved wild vine, Threeleaf cayratia • Hindi: *Amalbel, Gidardrak, Ramchana, Tamanya* • Marathi: *Ambatvel, Amboshi, Sarbarival* • Tamil: *Kattuppirantai* • Malayalam: *Amarcakkoti, Corivalli, Kattuperanta, Tsjori-valli, Vatakkoti* • Telugu: *Kanupu tige, Puli mada* • Kannada: *Heggoli* • Bengali: *Amal-lata* • Assamese: *Chepeta-lota* • Sanskrit: *Amlavetasah, Atyamlaparni, Gandirah*

Description:
Native to India, Bush Grape is a vine that climbs by means of tendrils which are found opposite the leaves.

The leaves are trifoliolate with petioles 2-3 cm long. The leaflets are ovate to oblong-ovate, 2-8 cm long, 1.5-5 cm wide, pointed at the tip, and coarsely toothed at the margins.

The flowers are small greenish white and borne on solitary cymes in leaf axils.

The fruit is fleshy, juicy, dark purple or black, nearly spherical and about 1 cm in diameter. Flowering: December.

Medicinal Uses:

The *root, ground with black pepper,* is applied *to boils.* The root is also used as an *astringent medicine.*

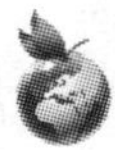

Shell Ginger

Botanical Name:

Alpinia zerumbet

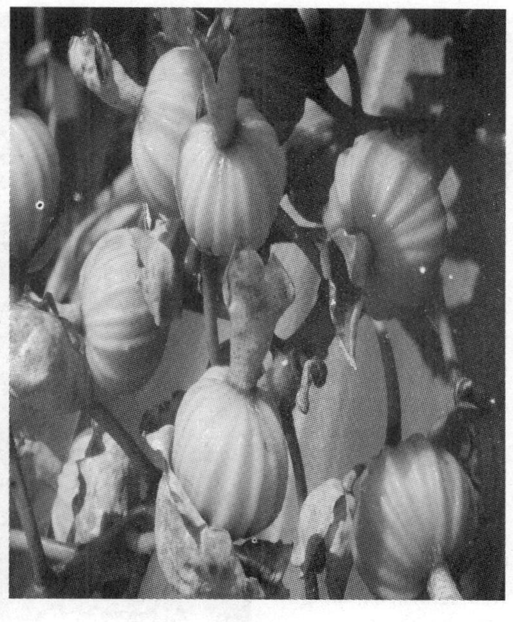

Family:

Zingiberaceae **(Ginger family)**

Common Names:

Shell Ginger, Light galangal, Pink porcelain lily • *Manipuri: Kanghoo* • Bengali: *Punnag champa*

Description:

Native to India, Shell ginger is a tall and dramatic landscape or container plant. The leaves are about 2 ft long and 6 in across and strikingly variegated with irregular stripes of green and yellow in some varieties. The habit is upright and does not require staking as do some other members of the ginger family. The flowers are white, tipped in pink, and borne in long pendant arches. In some varieties, there is no pink in the tip. The individual flowers are reminiscent of small seashells, which accounts for the Common Names "shell ginger". Typically, shell ginger grows to about 6 ft, but it can grow up to 12 ft high.

Medicinal Uses:

In Manipur, the *fresh rhizome* is applied to *ringworms* and other *skin diseases.* Rhizomes are *stimulant, carminative;* used in *rheumatism* and *bronchial catarrach.*

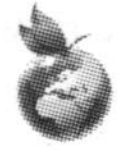

East Indian Arrowroot

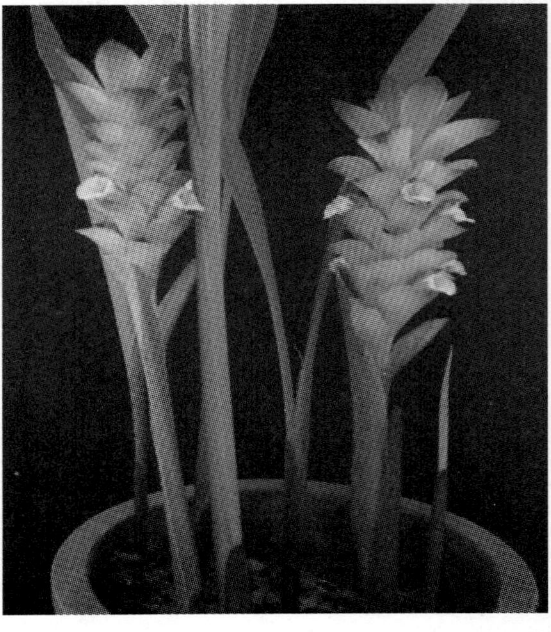

Botanical Name:
Curcuma angustifolia

Family:
Zingiberaceae **(Ginger family)**

Common Names:
East Indian Arrowroot, Bombay arrowroot • Hindi: *Tikhur* • Bengali: *Keturi halodhi* • Manipuri: *Yaipan* • Marathi: *Tavakeera, Tavakhira, Tavakila* • Malayalam: *Koova, Kuva-kizhanna* • Tamil: *Ararutkilangu, Kua, Ararut-kizhangu* • Kannadai: *Koove-hittu* • Telugu: *Ararut-gaddalu* • Sanskrit: *Tavakshira*

Description:
East Indian Arrowroot is an attractive ginger with stout underground rhizomes which lie dormant in winters.

In early spring, the flowers are produced before the leaves. Very colourful bracts make this a showy species. The shape and colour of the bracts are very variable.

The inflorescence lasts in full bloom on the plants for about three weeks and more. Good for cut flower use with a vase life of 10 days and more for fresh cut blooms.

Leaves grow to about 2ft tall and die down in autumn.

This species is found in the Eastern Himalays and inhabits bright open hillsides and woods. In Manipur, *pakodas* made using these flowers are considered a delicacy.

Medicinal Uses:

East Indian Arrowroot is recognised as *a medical herb.* It is *nutritive,* and is used as an *agreeable, non-irritating diet* in certain *chronic diseases,* during *convalescence from fevers,* in *irritations* of *the alimentary canal, pulmonary organs,* or of the urinary apparatus, and is well *suited for infants to supply the place of breast-milk,* or for a short time after having weaned them.

It may be given in the form of *jelly, variously seasoned with sugar, lemon-juice, fruit jellies, essences,* or *aromatics.*

Its jelly has no peculiar taste, and is less liable to become acidic in the stomach, and is generally preferred by young infants to all others, except *tapioca.*

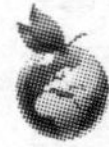

Wild Turmeric

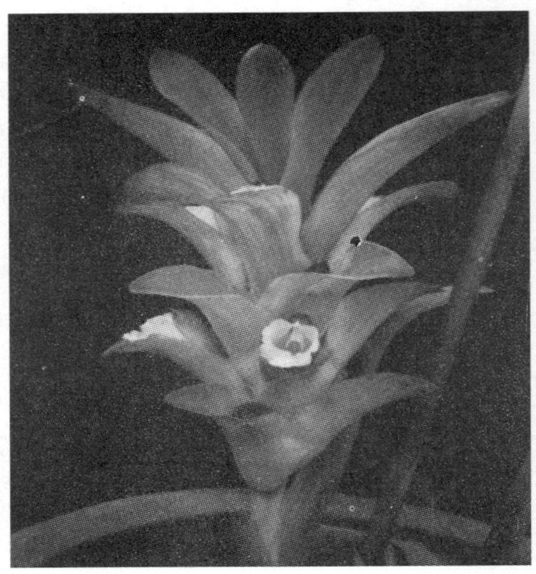

Botanical Name:

Curcuma aromatica

Family:

Zingiberaceae **(Ginger family)**

Common Names:

Wild turmeric, Aromatic turmeric • Hindi: *Jangli haldi* • Manipuri: *Lam Yaingang*
• Gujarati: *Zedoari*
• Tamil: *Kasturimanjal*
• Malayalam: *Kattumanna*
• Telugu: *Kasthuri Pasupa*
• Kannada: *Kasthuri Arishina*

Description:

Wild tumeric is an aromatic and pretty ginger with stout underground rhizomes. Foliage dies down in late in autumn and the rhizomes remain dormant in winter.

The inflorescence appears in early spring from the base of the rhizome. Flowers are pinkish white in colour, with an orange lip.

The stalk grows to about 8 to 10 inches tall, and is crowned with enlarged coloured bracts tipped with pink. Leaves appear after the flowers. When in full growth the plants can reach a height of about 3ft tall.

Leaves are broad and very decorative, elliptic, 3-4 ft long, and 20 cm wide, leaf-stalk being as long as the blade.

Good for cut-flower use with a vase life of about 10 days for a fresh stem. This species is found in the eastern Himalayas and inhabits warm forest areas.

Grows fast and vigorously during the summer monsoon months. Rhizomes used to a limited extent in villages for flavouring curries.

Medicinal Uses:

Wild turmeric is recognised as a medical herb with *strong antibiotic properties.*

It is believed to play a role in *preventing and curing cancer* in Chinese medicine. In an effort to remove cell accumulations, such as a *tumours and curcuma* is often utilised.

There are two species commonly used in *cancer therapy* that, like ginger, have a spicy taste.

It contains *aromatic volatile oils* that help to *remove excessive lipids from the blood, reduce aggregation of platelets* (sticking of the blood cells to form masses), and *reduce inflammation.*

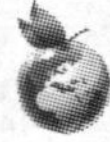

Black Turmeric

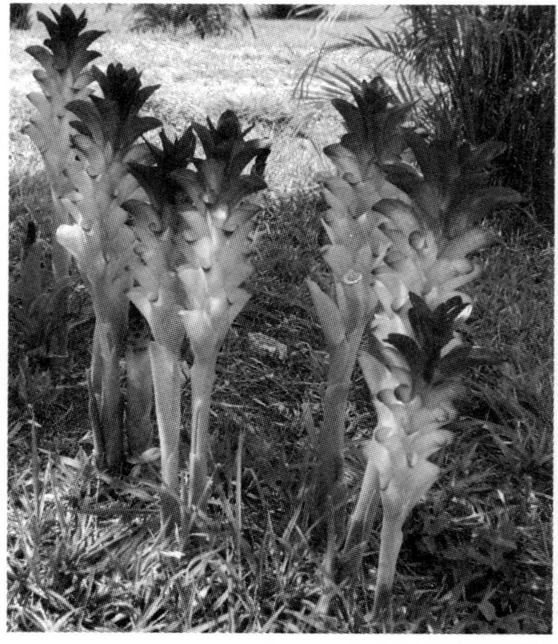

Botanical Name:
Curcuma caesia

Family:
Zingiberaceae **(Ginger family)**

Common Names:
Black Turmeric • Hindi: *Kali Haldi, Nar Kachura, Krishna kedar* • Manipuri: *Yaingang Amuba* • Marathi: *Kala-haldi* • Telugu: *Nalla Pasupu, Manupasupu* • Kannada: *Kariarishina, Naru kachora* • Bengali: *Kala haldi* • Mizo: *Aihang, Ailaihang* • Assamese: *Kala haladhi* • Nepali: *Kaalo haledo*

Description:
Black Turmeric is a perennial herb with bluish-black rhizome, native to North-East and Central India.

The leaves have a deep violet-red patch which runs through the length of the lamina. Usually, the upper side of the leaf is rough, velvety, but this character may vary.

Flowering bracts are green with a ferruginous tinge. Flower petals may be deep pink or red in colour. The rhizome is bitter, hot taste with pungent smell. Black Turmeric is used in Tantrik Sadhana.

The dried leaves are used as a source for fuel. Northern tribes use Black Turmeric as a talisman to keep the evil spirits away. Presently Black Turmeric is on the verge of extinction.

Medicinal Uses:

Claimed to be useful in treating *Piles, Leprosy, Bronchitis, Asthma, Cancer, Epilepsy, Fever, Wounds, Impotency, Fertility, Menstrual disorders, tooth ache, vomiting,* etc.

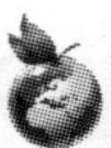

Turmeric

Botanical Name:
Curcuma longa

Family:
Zingiberaceae **(Ginger family)**

Common Names:
Turmeric • Assamese: *Halodhi* • Bengali: *Halud* • Gujarati: *Haldar* • Hindi: *Haldi* • Kannada: *Arishina, Arisina* • Malayalam: *Manjal* • Marathi: *Halad* • Nepali: *Haldi* • Oriya: *Haladi* • Sanskrit: *Haridra, Marmarii* • Tamil: *Manjal* • Telugu: *Haridra* • Urdu: *Haldi*

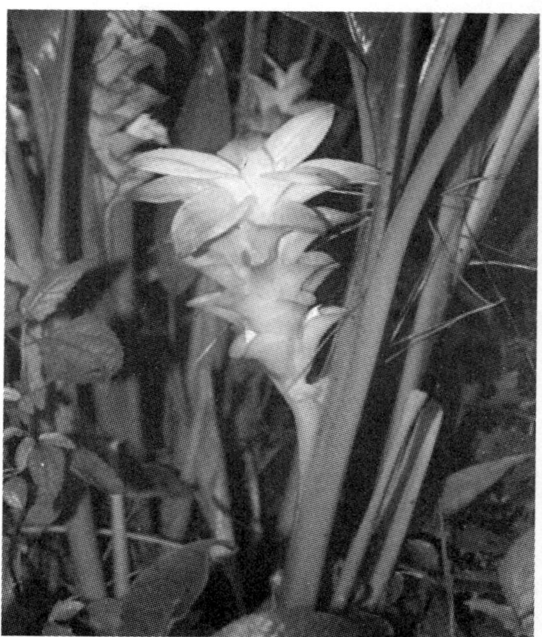

Description:
Turmeric is a rhizomatous herb, native to tropical South Asia. Turmeric is a very important spice in India, which produces nearly the whole world's crop and uses 80% of it. The plant grows to a height of 3-5 ft. It has oblong, pointed leaves and bears funnel-shaped yellow flowers, peeping out of large bracts. The rhizome is the portion of the plant used medicinally. It is usually boiled, cleaned, and dried, yielding a yellow powder. Dried Turmeric root is the source of the spice turmeric, the ingredient that gives curry powder its characteristic yellow colour.

Medicinal Uses:
Turmeric is used extensively in foods for both its *flavour and colour.* Turmeric has a long tradition of use in the *Chinese and Ayurvedic systems of medicine.*

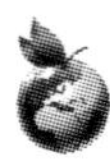

Hill Turmeric

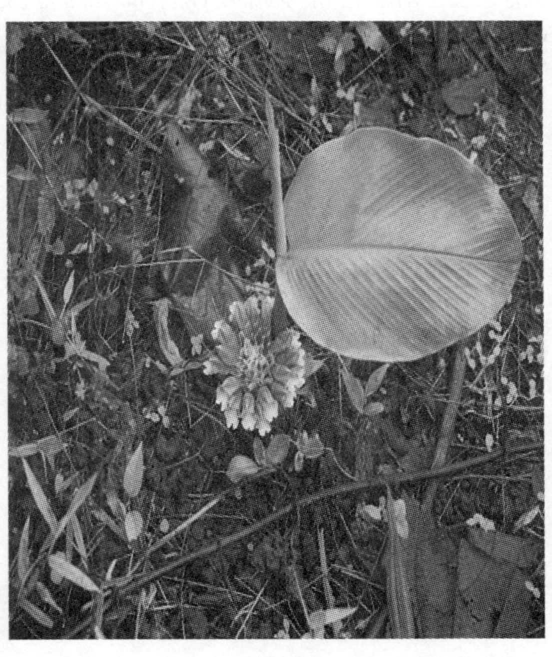

Botanical Name:

Curcuma pseudomontana

Family:

Zingiberaceae **(Ginger family)**

Common Names:

Hill Turmeric
• Hindi: *Kachura* • Marathi: *Raan halada, Shindalavana or Shindalavani*
• Tamil: *Kattu manjal*
• Malayalam: *Kattu manjal*

Description:

Hill Turmeric is an erect herb, growing to 75 cm tall, found on moist, shaded areas of wet forests and along sluggish grassy slopes of higher altitude.

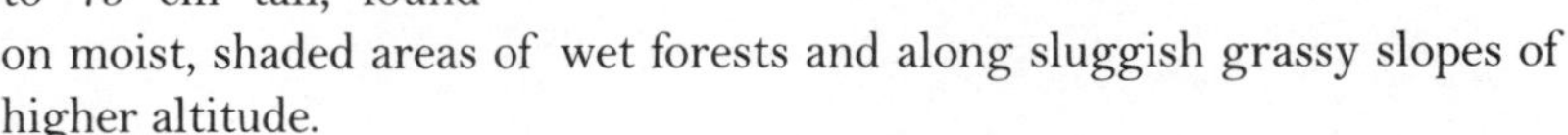

It has stout rootstock bearing small almond like sub-globose tubers at the ends of the fibrous roots. The tubers are fleshy and white inside, aromatic.

Leaves 3-5, oblong-lancelike, 20-30 x 6-9 cm, base acute, tip sharp, margin entire, hairless; shiny; leaf stalk and the leaf sheath up to 20 cm long.

Flowering spikes seen in the center of the previously formed tuft of leaves, 10-25 cm long, bearing numerous compactly arranged flowers; flowering bracts conspicuous, inverted egg shaped to lancelike, 3-5 x 1.5-2,cm, apex rounded to acute, hairless; green with a pink tip.

Non-flowering bracts (coma) oblong-lancelike, conspicuous, purple below and pinkish purple above.

Flowers 2-4 in each fertile bract, bright yellow, 3 cm long and 4 cm broad. Capsules spherical, splitting by 3-valves, smooth. Seeds ovoid or oblong, usually covered with arils. Flowering: June-September.

Medicinal Uses:

The *Savara tribes* in the *Eastern Ghats* of *Andhra Pradesh* use *tuber extracts* to cure *jaundice.*

The *Jatapu* and *Kaya tribes* apply *warm tuber paste* to treat *body swellings.* The women of Jatapu and Savara tribes eat *boiled tubers* to increase *lactation.*

The *Khand tribes* apply the *tuber paste* on the *head* for *cooling effect.*

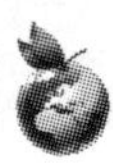

Red Ginger Lily

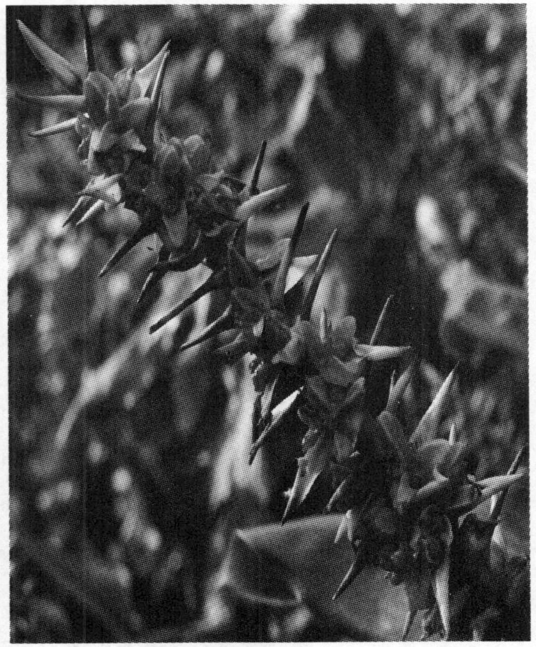

Botanical Name:
Hedychium marginatum

Family:
Zingiberaceae **(Ginger family)**

Common Names:
Red Ginger Lily
• Manipuri: *Takhellei angangba*

Description:
Red Ginger Lily is a very uncommon ginger with beautiful bright red flowers. In form, the flowers look similar to those of Butterfly Ginger Lily. Flowers appear in spikes. It is found in North-east India, particularly Manipur.

Medicinal Uses:
A *decoction of rhizomes* is given in *bronchitis* and *stomach complaints.*

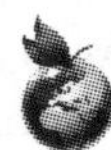

Spiked Ginger Lily

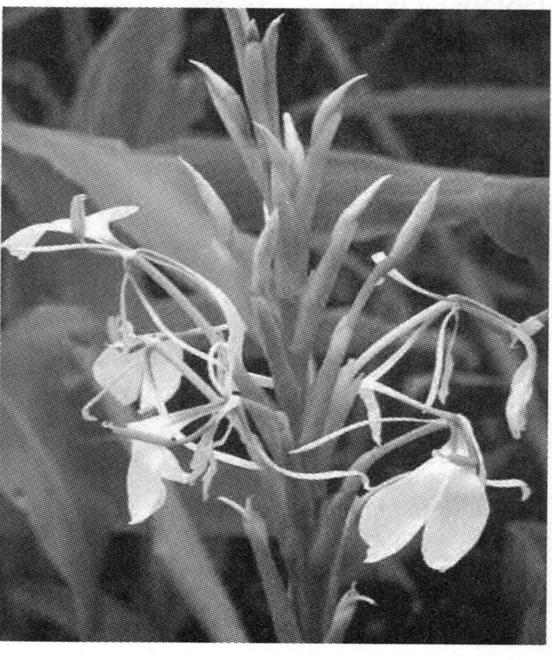

Botanical Name:

Hedychium spicatum

Family:

Zingiberaceae **(Ginger family)**

Common Names:

Spiked Ginger Lily
• Hindi: *Sandharlika, Kapur kachri*
• Manipuri: *Takhellei*
• Nepali: *Seto saro*

Description:

Spiked Ginger Lily is a smallish hardy ginger, growing to around 1-1.5 m, with leafy stems. Flowers are fragrant, white with an orange-red base, appearing in a dense spike, 15-25 cm, at the top of the stem. Flower tube is 5-6.5 cm long, much longer than the sepal cup, with white narrow petals spreading outwards. Lip is white with two elliptic lobes with an orange base. Filaments of the stamens are red. Leaves are oblong, up to a foot long and 4-12 cm broad, much like Haldi leaves. A perfume *Abeer* is obtained from the root stock. Spiked Ginger Lily is found from Himachal Pradesh to Arunachal Pradesh, at altitudes of 1800-2800 m. Flowering: July-August.

Medicinal Uses:

Rootstocks are used in *medicine.*

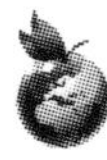

Puncture Vine

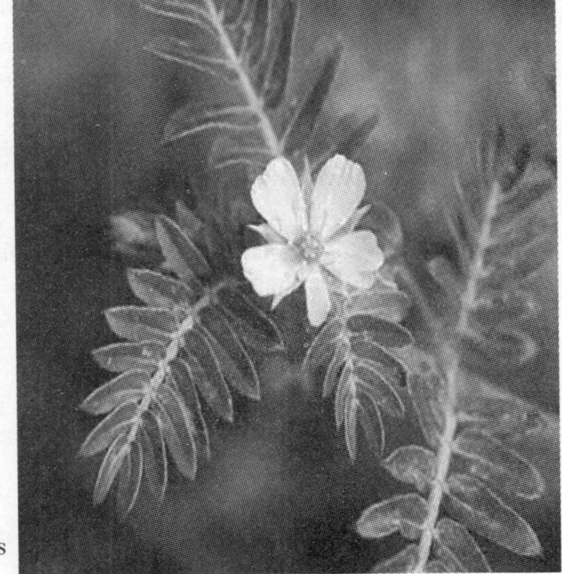

Botanical Name:

Tribulus terrestris

Family:

Zygophyllaceae
(Caltrop family)

Common Names:

Puncture Vine, Caltrop, Yellow Vine, Goathead • Hindi: *Gokharu* • Urdu: *Gokhru* • Bengali: *Gokhru kanta* • Telugu: *Cinnpalleru* • Tamil: *Palleru-mullu* • Malayalam: *Nerinnii*

Description:

This is an obnoxious weed, whose seeds are incredibly painful to step on, they easilly puncture your bicycle tires, and sometimes have to be pulled out of your pets' paws.

It is a tap-rooted herbaceous perennial plant that grows as a summer annual in colder climates. The stems radiate from the crown to a diameter of about 10 cm to over 1 m, often branching.

They are usually prostrate, forming flat patches, though they may grow more upwards in shade or among taller plants.

The leaves are pinnately compound with leaflets less than a quarter-inch long. The flowers are 4-10 mm wide, with five lemon-yellow petals.

A week after each flower blooms, it is followed by a fruit that easily falls apart into four or five single-seeded nutlets.

The nutlets or "seeds" are hard and bear two sharp spines, 10 mm long and 4-6 mm broad point-to-point.

These nutlets strikingly resemble goats' or bulls' heads; the 'horns' are sharp enough to puncture bicycle tyres and to cause considerable pain to unshod feet.

Medicinal Uses:

Tribulus is mentioned in *ancient Indian Ayurvedic medical texts* dating back thousands of years. Tribulus has been widely used in the *Ayurvedic system of medicine* for the treatment of *sexual dysfunction* and various *urinary disorders.*

The Greeks used Tribulus Terrestris as *a diuretic.* In China and Vietnam, it has been used in the *treatment of post-partum hemorrhage, epistaxis* and *gastro-intestinal bleeding.*

Tribulus terrestris is being promoted as a *testosterone booster* for the purpose of *building muscles* and *increasing sex drive.*

It does not work like DHEA and *androstenedione* 100, which are *progenitors* of *testosterone.* Instead, claims have been made that it enhances the testosterone levels by increasing the luteinising hormone levels.

V&S OLYMPIAD SERIES FOR CLASSES 1-10

MATHS OLYMPIAD (CLASS 1-10)

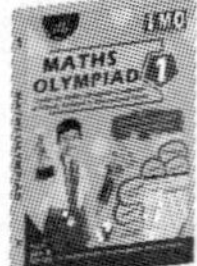
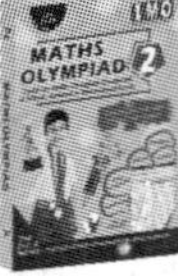
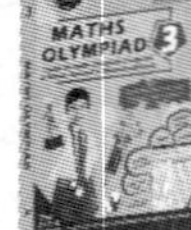
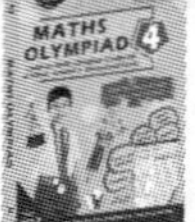
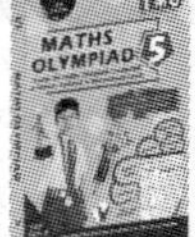
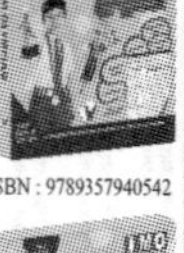

ISBN : 9789357940504 ISBN : 9789357940511 ISBN : 9789357940528 ISBN : 9789357940535 ISBN : 9789357940542

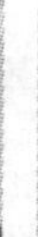
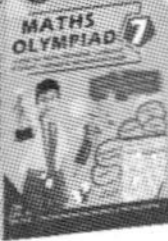
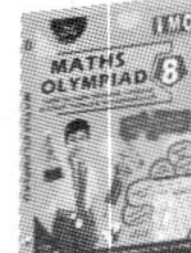
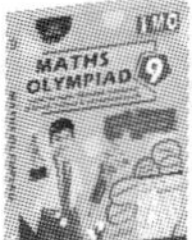

ISBN : 9789357940559 ISBN : 9789357940566 ISBN : 9789357940573 ISBN : 9789357940580 ISBN : 9789357940597

SCIENCE OLYMPIAD (CLASS 1-10)

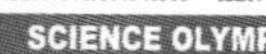
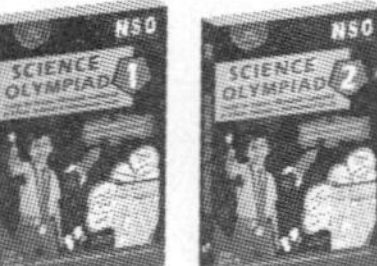
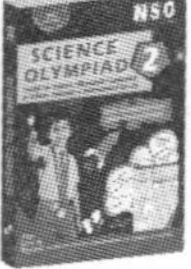
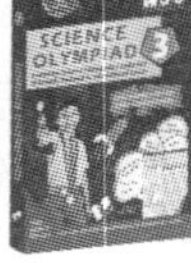
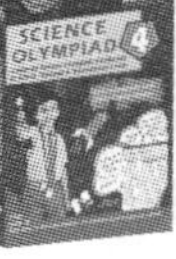
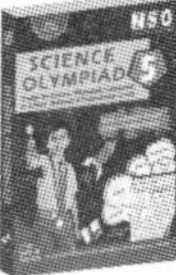

ISBN : 9789357940405 ISBN : 9789357940412 ISBN : 9789357940429 ISBN : 9789357940436 ISBN : 9789357940443

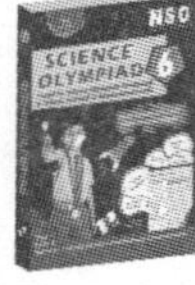
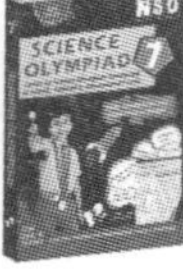
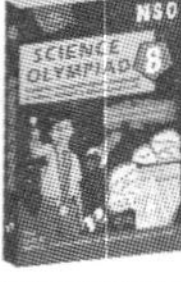
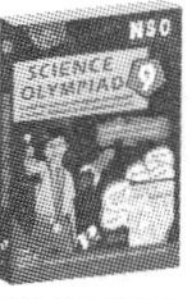
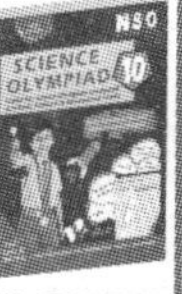

ISBN : 9789357940450 ISBN : 9789357940467 ISBN : 9789357940474 ISBN : 9789357940481 ISBN : 9789357940498

CYBER OLYMPIAD (CLASS 1-10)

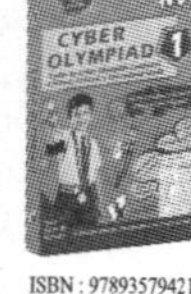
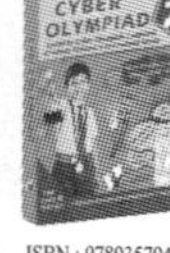
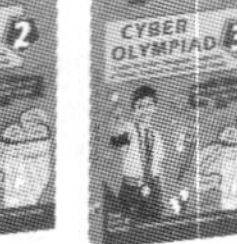
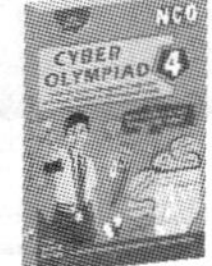
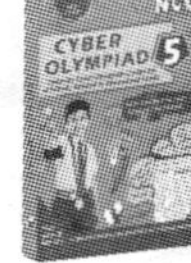

ISBN : 9789357942102 ISBN : 9789357940603 ISBN : 9789357940610 ISBN : 9789357940627 ISBN : 9789357940634

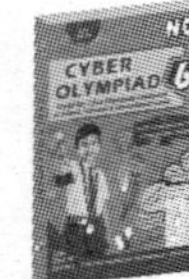
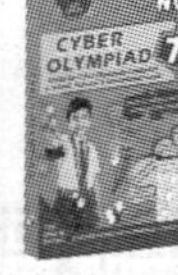
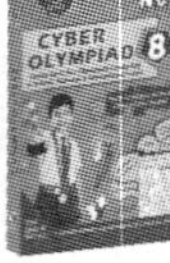
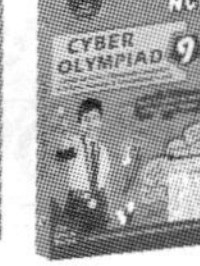
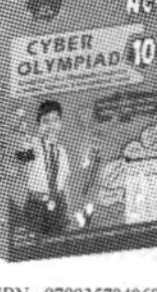

ISBN : 9789357940641 ISBN : 9789357940658 ISBN : 9789357940665 ISBN : 9789357940672 ISBN : 9789357940689

ENGLISH OLYMPIAD (CLASS 1-10)

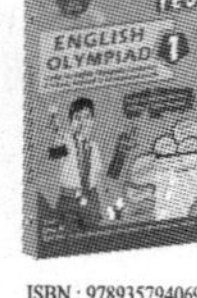

ISBN : 9789357940696 ISBN : 9789357940702 ISBN : 9789357940719 ISBN : 9789357940726 ISBN : 9789357940733

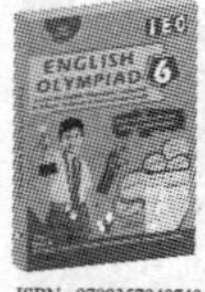
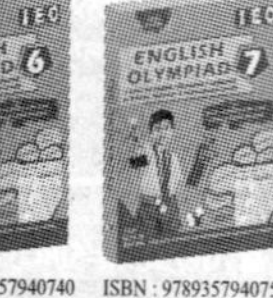
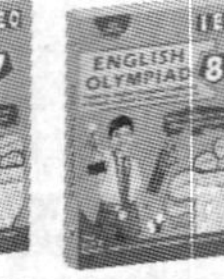
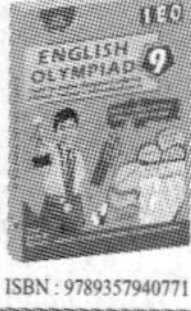

ISBN : 9789357940740 ISBN : 9789357940757 ISBN : 9789357940764 ISBN : 9789357940771 ISBN : 9789357940788

OLYMPIAD SAMPLE PAPER (CLASS 1-10)

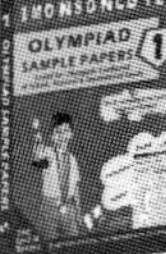
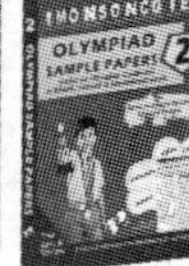
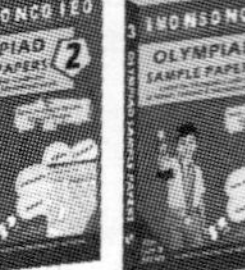
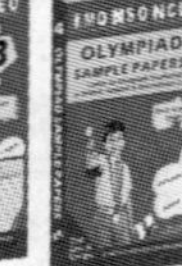
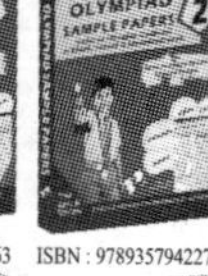
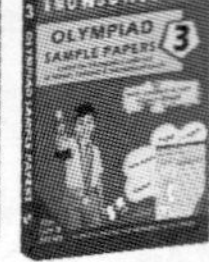
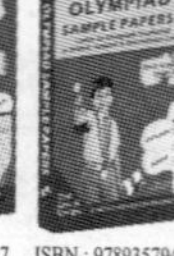

ISBN : 9789357942263 ISBN : 9789357942270 ISBN : 9789357942287 ISBN : 97893579422

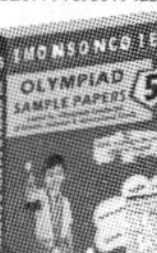
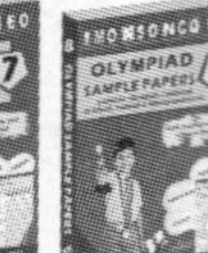

ISBN : 9789357942300 ISBN : 9789357942317 ISBN : 9789357942324 ISBN : 97893579423

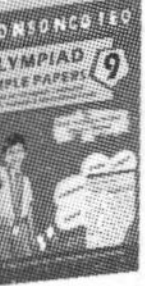
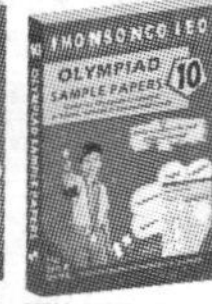
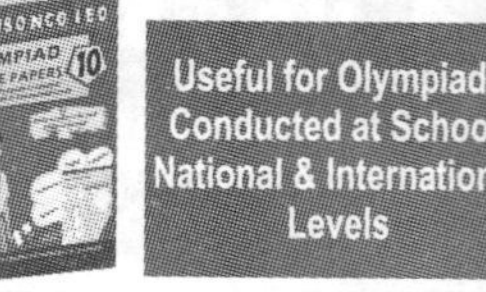

ISBN : 9789357942348 ISBN : 9789357942355

Useful for Olympiads Conducted at School, National & Internationa Levels

OLYMPIAD COMBO PACK (4 BOOK SET)

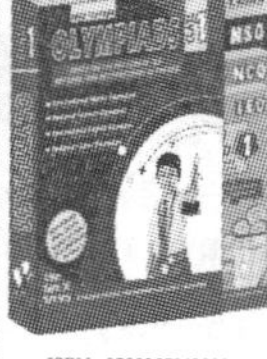
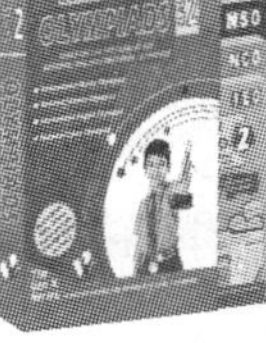
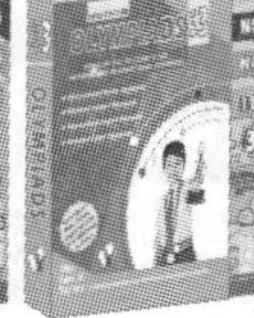

ISBN : 9789357942003 ISBN : 9789357942010 ISBN : 9789357942027

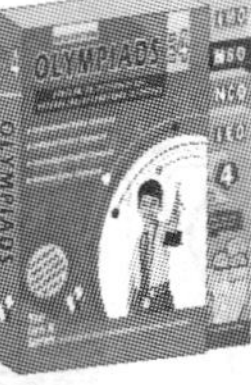
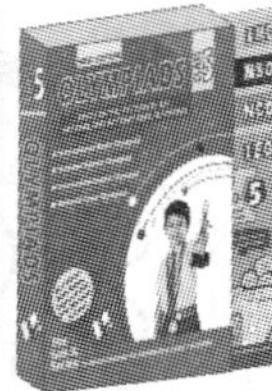
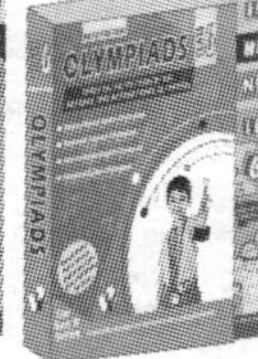

ISBN : 9789357942034 ISBN : 9789357942041 ISBN : 9789357942058

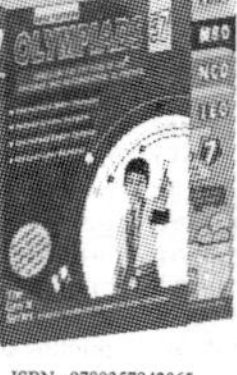
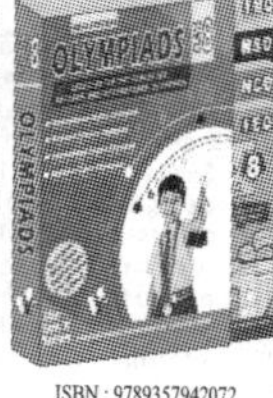
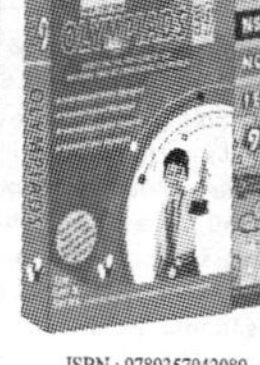

ISBN : 9789357942065 ISBN : 9789357942072 ISBN : 9789357942089

ISBN : 9789357942096

CLASS 1-10 ENGLISH, MATHS, CYBER, SCIENCE OLYMPIAD 4 BOOKS SAVER COMBO PACK